TESTIMONIALS

If you talk to most Americans today, the majority of them want to lose weight. Many will tell you that they are ready to do something about it now. In fact, some of them desperately feel the need to take action but hardly know where to begin. They talk about trying to juggle too many tasks; about having too many time-consuming responsibilities such as managing a home, a business or a career, attending to their children's needs and schedules, and about not having enough time to prepare proper meals. Today's typical Americans feel pressured, unfulfilled, frustrated about their weight, and too tired to live a healthy life.

Years of experience have proven my weight loss methodology to be successful. I believe the success is due to my understanding that most people lack the confidence to change their eating habits on their own. People need motivation in order to follow a diet. Whenever I encounter a new patient, my first goal is to treat that person with the respect he or she deserves for making the effort to change. The atmosphere of respect encourages patients to relax and tell me about themselves, their relationship with food, their health concerns, and any other problems they might be facing. Next, I use dialogue to create a positive relationship, which encourages trust and open communication. Once the patient relaxes and opens up to my advice, I am then able to advise him or her about changing dietary habits. Throughout the relationship, I try to build up a patient's self-confidence until the patient reaches the point of believing in his or her own ability to create positive lifestyle change.

One of my most striking memories of a patient's long-term success is that of a woman named Elaine. When she first came to my clinic several years ago, she was overweight, pale and anxious. The signs of fatigue were visible on her face. She complained about stomach gas, bloatedness, pain, and constipation. Additionally, she experienced great difficulty sleeping at night. Within only one month of following a high fiber-low fat diet she reported feeling energetic, she no longer had symptoms of digestive distress, and her skin condition improved dramatically. In fact, she glowed with vitality; a more positive person; and a new woman. She lost 22-pounds and felt great. The following letter is from my patient, Elaine.

"Passion inspires richness and depth to your daily living. Dr. Tooshi triggers the passion to improve your life, get healthy, and live life with zest. The diet adds balance to your well being. I have achieved all of this after 50 years of being miserable about my weight. Dr. Tooshi is my anchor."

—Elaine S.

"A weight loss program tailor-made to your individual needs with food you like to eat. No pills, no exercise, no excuses … just amazing results. Dr. Tooshi is truly the WIZARD OF WEIGHT LOSS!"

—Nick Coppola,
Greenworks Environmental, LLC Wall, NJ

"Dr. Alan Tooshi not only changed my life, he also changed the life of all my friends and family that I recommended to go and see him. It's been almost two and a half years, and still my weight is off. Seeing is believing. If you have a real weight problem, I strongly recommend you see him if you really want to lose weight. He truly changed my life.
Thank you Dr. Tooshi for giving me a New Me."

—Arthur Gentile, Manalapan, N.J.
Top Catch, Inc., Brooklyn, N.Y.

"For years I've tried to lose weight and due to medical problems, the pounds never came off. I tried Dr. Tooshi's nutritional program, and found not only did

I lose weight, but also my health and attitude improved and I lost the weight I wanted to. I am still on his program and will follow it faithfully."

—Barbara R.

"I am honored to write this for a man I hold dear. In April of 2007 I walked into the office of Dr. Tooshi, Ph.D. I was privileged to also meet his beautiful wife Diane, who gave me an overview of what was to unfold before me. The day I walked into their office I was sad, depressed, negative, grossly overweight and figured "why not … I'll try another diet" … little did I know the life changing experience about to unfold before me. What I received, thanks to Dr. Tooshi, was a knowledge of my own body; learning how foods work in my body; learning about <u>why</u> I eat, not just <u>what</u> I eat; and learning how to begin to save my own life. A whole new world opened up for me. I lost weight; I gained confidence; I unburdened myself of many emotional issues; I gained a positive outlook from Dr. Tooshi that no one had ever given me; and I became a <u>healthy</u>, happy woman again. I got a **LIFESTYLE CHANGE**. My husband joined the "Tooshi Train" in June of 2007 and has also enjoyed tremendous success. Dr. Tooshi brings with him a wealth of knowledge, an amazing, kind and caring nature, an expertise on foods and their chemical make-up, and a positive outlook on life that is contagious. We are so honored to have Dr. Tooshi and Diane in our lives. It is now late December 2008 and my husband, Rick and I have lost over 100 pounds collectively. We have gained the knowledge of a **GIANT** … Dr. Alan Tooshi."

—With love and thanks,
Renee and Rick Narson, Freehold, NJ

"It is difficult to know where to begin writing the countless ways that Dr. Tooshi has helped me and others like me. I first met Dr. Tooshi in June of 2003. I have the pleasure of seeing him twice a week since that time. After Dr. Tooshi's diet helped me get rid of thirty pounds, I started working for him as his receptionist. For that reason I have seen him assist people in changing their lives. His diet is successful in weigh loss. His diet has helped people with all ranges of medical conditions from high blood pressure and cholesterol to diabetes and irritable bowel syndrome and many more conditions. I would have to say the biggest change I see in people is in their mind. Of course physically they look different, but they are happier, more confident, more outgoing and their self-esteem sores. Physically one can see the changes in the people, but they also have other physical benefits that one cannot see. People have expressed to me how they sleep better; they have more energy, their skin and hair look and feel better. Women have expressed how the side effects of their menstrual cycle are better. Many patients have told me that their knees and backs no longer hurt. The list goes on and on."

—Debi Richards
Marlboro, NJ

FAT AMERICA

FAT AMERICA

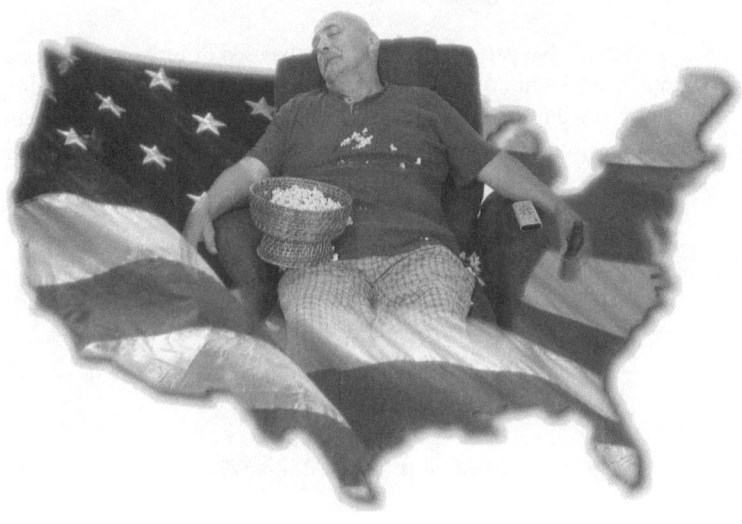

◆

Change your lifestyle

Dr. Alan M. Tooshi, Ph.D.

iUniverse, Inc.
New York Lincoln Shanghai

FAT AMERICA
Change your lifestyle

Copyright © 2008 by Alan M. Tooshi

iUniverse books may be ordered through booksellers or by contacting:

iUniverse
2021 Pine Lake Road, Suite 100
Lincoln, NE 68512
www.iuniverse.com
1-800-Authors (1-800-288-4677)

Because of the dynamic nature of the Internet, any Web addresses or links contained in this book may have changed since publication and may no longer be valid.

You should not undertake any diet/exercise regimen recommended in this book before consulting your personal physician. Neither the author nor the publisher shall be responsible or liable for any loss or damage allegedly arising as a consequence of your use or application of any information or suggestions contained in this book.

ISBN: 978-0-595-47811-8 (pbk)
ISBN: 978-0-595-71430-8 (cloth)

Printed in the United States of America

It is with the deepest appreciation; I wish to thank the people who came to my clinic believing in me. I am always inspired by their motivation and dedication. It is through our effort I have found my mission in life: to help those who are trying to free themselves from the physical and emotional pain of being overweight.

I wish to thank Michelle Alaia, Pat Lazar, and Debi Richards for their effort in completing the manuscript for this book and my first book, "Dr. Tooshi's High Fiber Diet."

I would like to thank my son, Michael and my wife, Diane, for their love and support and work in editing the manuscript.

I would especially like to thank Renee Narson for trusting my ideas, sharing her story, and embracing life again. Her success and joyfulness gives me tremendous professional and personal satisfaction. Thank you for your courage, strength, and dedication.

In conclusion, I would like to pay tribute to my two dogs Wolfie, a Samoyed and Baby Duke, a Pug who sat at my feet, followed my footsteps, and kept me company through many months of writing and exercising. They are my "silent partners" in this effort.

Contents

Part V   *RECIPES FOR HEALTH AND LONGEVITY*

PREFACE

Most people may not be ready to accept my proposal but I am convinced that lifestyle choices are the root cause of our nation's health problems. Stress, overeating and the lack of physical fitness have resulted in an American obesity epidemic. Today sixty-five percent (65%) of adults and forty percent (40%) of children in the United States are overweight. As long as we persevere without changing our lifestyles, we will continue to be plagued by stress, medical problems and fatigue. My solution will undoubtedly cause you to reexamine your values and your relationship with food. It is my purpose to encourage you to change your beliefs about stress, proper nutrition, and exercise and to challenge your perspective on disease and aging.

America needs a wake-up call. The twin forces of stress and poor eating habits have cast a dismal shadow over our future—our lives are in jeopardy. Yet, we can stop destroying ourselves and our children's future by mustering the conviction to change. We have a choice to make. The power, desire, and ability to make the right choice lies within each of us. First, we must recognize that our habits are unhealthy. Next, we need to examine the options: either we do nothing or we take the opportunity to get informed and assume control of our lives by applying the lessons that we learn.

We will not find a long-term solution for chronic disease, namely heart disease, cancer, diabetes, and stroke unless we change our outlook and take back responsibility for our lives. Despite having the best medicine, medical treatment and technology in history, Americans are less healthy today than they were fifty years ago. We can no longer afford to relegate the responsibility for our health to the medical professionals and pharmaceutical companies.

I believe that the goal of public health is to improve our quality of life without endangering our environment. We must value our health just as much as we value our economic well being. Fundamental progress in public health depends upon resolving the major health problems that face our nation today. The environment that we have become accustomed to since the end of the Second World War is damaging our quality of life. It has made us vulnerable to diseases that did not pose a significant threat in the past such as cancer, heart disease, stroke, diabetes, and obesity. The changes, which have occurred in American society since the end of World War II amount to nothing short of a revolution. Post-World War II America is characterized by drastic changes in the eating habits and life-styles of American families. Each generation is becoming more obsessed with dieting and relieving our high-stressed way of life.

Today, we invest billions of dollars in research efforts aimed at finding phar-maceutical solutions to our health and weight problems. Instead, we must seek out a solution by addressing the root causes. Prescription drugs and fad diets have not provided a satisfactory remedy as the number of people afflicted by such ail-ments is rising year after year.

Our current health care system focuses on intervention. What we need is a method that makes prevention the top priority. The best way to begin any life-style change is by gaining more information and a better understanding of per-sonal health. A good education will help you to select proper food and engage in daily physical activities. With this book I hope to share my knowledge, wisdom, and understanding about the physiological benefits of a healthy diet and life-style and regular exercise.

Part One of the book is devoted to explaining the root causes of obesity in America. In Part Two, I discuss the role that nutrition plays in health and well-being. Part Three explains the physiological benefits of exercise. In Part Four, I've presented a more technical discussion about the effects that exercise can have on the cardiovascular system and on the respiratory system. Part Four will provide individuals who may not have studied biology or human physiology with the knowledge necessary to understand how those systems function. These technical discussions are derived from the 20-minute lectures that made such a difference to the "exercise and lecture group" from my research at New Jersey City University. Additionally, in Part Five, I have included some of my best recipes in order to help the reader select a proper diet. Finally, I hope this book will help anyone desiring to make the necessary lifestyle changes in order to ensure a healthier hap-pier future.

ABOUT THE AUTHOR

Dr. Alan M. Tooshi taught Public Health Nutrition, Weight Control, Environmental Health, Mental Health, and Research Methodology at New Jersey City University for thirty-three years. He has been a keynote speaker and lecturer to many civic organizations, including the Rotary and Lions Clubs. His lectures focus on weight-loss through diet and exercise with a particular emphasis on the relationship between nutrition and mental health. Since 1979 he has organized diets for private patients with chronic health problems such as diabetes, high blood pressure, heart disease, digestive ailments and for those who just want to lose weight without using pills or eating packaged food.

Several years ago Dr. Tooshi conducted an exercise program at the New Jersey City University. The purpose of the program was to study the effects of physical exercise on body-weight, blood pressure and cholesterol. Forty businesspeople from local communities participated. He divided them into two groups: an "exercise only group" and an "exercise and lecture group." The exercise group worked out in the gym for forty-five minute sessions, three days a week. By contrast, the exercise and lecture group received twenty-minute lectures immediately before their forty-five minute workout. The lectures included topics such as the effects of exercise on circulation, metabolism, blood pressure, and cholesterol, as well as stress reduction. The exercise only group frequently complained about exercise being too hard, too boring, or else they reported tiring easily. As the study progressed, this group did not show consistent attendance at the exercise sessions. Nearly everyone had an excuse for missing sessions.

The exercise and lecture group demonstrated a different attitude. In the gym they performed with tremendous energy, showing enthusiasm and rarely complaining. Their attendance was near perfect and many told him that they continued exercising on their own. As a result of the study, he concluded that the reason for the "exercise and lecture" group's successful performance was due to their understanding of the benefits that exercise offers one's health and emotional well-being. The "exercise only" group completed the program with the same information they had when started. In actuality, they did not succeed because they never changed their thinking.

Dr. Tooshi believes the current rise in obesity lies in the public's lack of knowledge about the consequences of poor dietary habits and lifestyles. Today's occurring rates of heart disease, stroke, diabetes, and cancer provide sufficient evidence. The majority of diets fail to produce meaningful results because patients fail to change their eating habits and lifestyles. Consequently, Dr. Tooshi is convinced that diet plans by themselves without education and counseling can never solve the nation's obesity crisis.

In October of 1979 Dr. Tooshi opened his diet clinic and developed his individualized diet program providing vital information to the patients about the risks of obesity and the role of proper nutrition in preventing heart disease, stroke, diabetes, and blood pressure. Ever since, his program has become successful, with a very low drop out rate among patients. Most patients who lost weight have managed to keep it off for years and have changed the way they think about food, abandoning their former unhealthy habits. Based on his many years of experience working with students and patients, he believes that we cannot win the struggle against obesity in America unless we change our lifestyles.

PART I
FAT AMERICA

1

THE RISE OF OBESITY

Obesity has become an epidemic in America. It is responsible for more than five million deaths each year and plays a major role in the rise of heart disease, cancer, diabetes, high blood pressure, and stroke. Today, more than sixty-five percent of adults and forty percent of children are overweight in America. Our overweight population is increasing year by year despite the increasing numbers of people trying to lose weight. The burden on our health care system for treating obesity costs over a billion dollars annually. The book's primary goal is to provide the public with the information it needs in order to prevent and defeat obesity in the United States. By the explanations and information I provide in this book, you will be able to make wiser choices regarding your diet and lifestyle. The next time you visit your doctor he or she may be surprised to find that your blood pressure, blood sugar, cholesterol levels, and body weight are more under control mainly because you changed your lifestyle and eating habits. The truth of the matter is that lifestyle change involves three things—changing your food intake, changing your physical activity pattern, and better stress management planning. The challenge America faces is in accepting individual responsibility for our health and that obesity and weight gain is caused by our overeating, poor selection of foods, lack of regular exercise, and our inability to manage emotional stress.

Currently the average American's caloric intake is very high, almost twice that of Europeans. A typical person requires approximately 1,500 calories per day. The average American consumes about 3,000 calories a day, yet their diet is considered to be poor by nutritional standards. The average American diet consists of fried foods, fast-foods, red meats, pastry items, starchy foods and very little fruits, vegetables, and seafood. Regular physical exercise plays a very important role in weight loss. Exercise helps increase metabolic rate, burn fat, lower blood pressure, and strengthen circulation. Most American's are poor at managing emotional stress. They turn to food for comfort and to release their tension. Unfortunately, they turn to foods that are high in fat, sugar, and salt. Stress is a major factor in the causes of obesity in our culture. The average American will consume more than 1,000 calories a day from the snack food industry. It is no wonder life feels like an emotional roller coaster and rates of depression are on the rise.

Many people believe that obesity is caused by genetic factors rather than by overeating. Yet, if we examine the history of American culture and eating habits, we will come to the conclusion that there is little support for the connection between genetics and obesity. The people who left the continent of Europe for a new life in America, found a beautiful land with magnificent and majestic mountains, rivers, lakes and valleys, with breathtaking sunrises and sunsets. But life was not easy; it involved clearing the land, cultivating, building homes, raising cattle, and raising families. People worked very hard, but at the end of the day they gathered around the dinner table to enjoy homemade food and discuss the days events with each other. Life was simpler then in respect to family roles. Women mainly stayed at home raising children. They cooked and took care of the home. Men chiefly worked in the fields and factories to put the food on the table. Some children helped at home with the chores or went to school. There was a productive partnership between husbands, wives, and children because each of them accepted their role within the family structure. Obesity was not a problem in those days. There were no overweight people in the working class community. Overweight people were found chiefly among the affluent members of society who typically consumed more food and did very little physical work. Overweight women were often idolized in paintings and popular culture due to their scarcity among the general populace. Their pictures were posted in taverns and public places, very similar to our glorification of contemporary skinny fashion models.

The majority of the population—men, women and children—were very healthy, trim, rugged, and strong. Diseases such as heart disease, cancer, diabetes, high blood pressure, stroke and digestive disorders were seldom seen among them. Their good health was attributed to their diet, physical activity and lack of daily stress. Even up to the beginning of World War II, Americans did not have much incidence of obesity. We must understand that we are the descendants of those people. To say that obesity is genetic is inaccurate. Obesity is based mainly on overeating, lack of physical activity, and stress.

After World War II, when soldiers returned home, they got married and took higher paying jobs because of America's economic boom. Industries and factories increased their production and all kinds of goods and services became available to people. Life became easier with newfound income and purchasing power. People enjoyed better services, more food, and better housing. Women entered the workforce. They left the home to work alongside of men. Now that husbands and wives worked outside the home, mothers were left with very little time for cooking and caring for the house and children. In 1954, the TV dinner was invented saving women time by allowing them to just put such products in the oven for 20 minutes and serving it to the whole family.

In 1960, fast food stores came into being. At the same time many new eating establishments were opening. The new restaurants, diners, and fast-food vendors designed menus with attractive pictures, encouraging people to eat more for a reasonable cost. These establishments offered food high in fat, salt, and additives. The consumption of these foods gradually gave rise to obesity and major diseases. Restaurants and fast food chains replaced the family dining table. Family members had very little opportunity to discuss the important events of the day among themselves. Both wife and husband worked all day and left the supervision of children to others. At the end of the day many parents arrived home, tired and stressed with little energy for anything other than watching television and eating. Full-time employment and household responsibilities coupled with caring for children created stress and dissatisfaction within families. The resulting stress gradually contributed increasing instances of separation, divorce and single-parenthood. In order to ease the stress and frustration, people turned to food for comfort. Lack of daily exercise and overeating led American men, women and children to obesity. Therefore a relationship between food and stress reveals a dependence upon eating as a source of pleasure.

As obesity increased in America, the drug manufacturers found the disease to be a goldmine. They began producing a variety of pills and drugs and marketing weight loss as a quick, easy method to achieve good health. Additionally, the medical profession cashed in by offering people ways to lose weight through stomach surgery and liposuction. At the same time many diet books, pills, high protein diets, low-calorie diets, a grapefruit diet, and eat-all-you-want diets promised Americans a solution to their weight problems. Such products, books, and pills had a very modest and temporary effect on the rising epidemic.

Other companies took advantage of this phenomenon and manufacturing various exercise gadgets and equipment designed for weight-loss. Many of them claimed that five to ten minutes of daily exercise would help people lose fat from their hips, thighs, buttocks, and abdomen. People with questionable research backgrounds in nutrition and exercise wrote the diet books and magazine articles that claim to help people lose weight. Such authors never graduated from college with a degree in nutrition nor exercise physiology. Even many medical doctors have written books about nutrition without sufficient training in that field because we know that most medical schools do not offer nutrition courses as part of their normal curriculum. Weight loss centers also opened and profited from the general lack of awareness. They offered frozen foods, prepackaged high fat, high salt meals, and rich snacks. Few, if any, of the diet programs and other products have succeeded in arresting the ever-increasing number of obese people in America.

Obesity has risen tremendously over the last twenty years. I believe very strongly that nothing will help to reduce obesity until people modify their lifestyle. The lifestyle changes necessarily involve: developing new eating habits, participating in daily exercise, and reducing emotional stress. The road to successful habit change is through education; it is through our thoughts. Only through education can we understand the importance of health and well being. By participating in exercise, eating a proper diet and coping with stress we can find the solution to our national health epidemic.

The purpose of this book is to discuss in detail the physiological benefits of exercise and its effect on the cardiovascular system, metabolism, energy, and muscular strength. The second section deals with the function and requirement of carbohydrates, proteins, fats, vitamins and minerals and their effects on the immune system, circulation, and digestive system. In addition, I describe how to select a proper diet, lose weight and maintain it.

Causes of Obesity

Obesity is one of the major health problems facing people today. It is a breeding ground for many of our health problems, especially heart disease, diabetes, cancer, high blood pressure, high cholesterol and stroke. The rate of obesity is increasing year by year. Today over sixty-five percent (65%) of American adults are classified as either overweight or obese. The treatment for obesity related illness costs billions of dollars each year.

Overeating and lack of physical activity cause obesity. It has very little connection to genetics at all. Genetically, people are born with three body types all over the world.
They are:

1. Ectomorphic—Slim, skinny but not physically strong. This group makes up five to eight percent of the world population.

2. Mesomorphic—Muscular, strong, very healthy people. This group makes up eighty to eighty-eight percent of the world population.

3. Endomorphic—Overweight, susceptible to illness, shorter life span. This group makes up five to eight percent of the world population.

If we compare five to eight percent genetic obesity with sixty-five percent actual obesity rates, we will conclude that the overweight problem in America has no relationship to genetic obesity. Obesity today is caused by over consumption of food and sedentary living. I call it environmental obesity, not genetic obesity. Sixty years ago, obesity was not a major problem in America. There were very few overweight people and those who were overweight were among the wealthy and highly active social groups. They consumed more food and were less physically active than their working class counterparts. After 1950, when the economic system improved, a large number of women entered the workforce. Eating outside the home increased tremendously. Women no longer had the time to prepare meals at home and some couples worked longer hours. Eating out became a necessary function of this new lifestyle as well as a symbol of affluence. Food establishments popped up everywhere opening up an avenue of variety with affordability. This choice came with a price. Restaurant foods were high in calories, fats, salt, and chemical additives. In some cases, people began taking home precooked meals. Activity levels began to shift from active to sedentary, contributing to the rise in obesity. To combat environmental obesity we must do the following:

• Prepare more meals at home

• Consume more fruits and vegetables

• Eat more seafood

• Reduce consumption of saturated fats

• Reduce consumption of red meats

• Reduce consumption of non-complex carbohydrates such as pasta, muffins, pie, cake, and soft drinks

• Reduce salt intake by substituting spices and by ordering grilled seafoods or chicken with vegetables when dining out.

• Increase physical activity by adding regular exercise to your weekly routine (see chapter on exercise).

Childhood Obesity

Today there is much concern about epidemic levels of childhood obesity. More than forty-five percent of American children are overweight, with many being obese. In the past, it was a rarity to see an obese child among those playing in the neighborhood, parks, or schoolyard. Previously children's diets were more nutritious because they were cooked and eaten at home with the family. Good eating habits were shared and learned. Today, a child's lifestyle has shifted to coincide with the busy lifestyle of parents. In general, children exercise less and eat more fast foods. Schools offer team sports in gym rather than the more rigorous military based program of the past where children ran obstacle courses, climbed and did calisthenics. In team sports, there is less active participation per class period because participants generally move only when the ball comes their way. For the most part gym classes involve stop and go activity rather than sustained activity.

After school, a majority of children spend time on the computer playing games or talking on-line. Oftentimes computer activity is paired with snack foods, soft drinks or microwave mini meals. Most parents are working when children arrive home from school or just do not have the time to prepare a nutritious after school snack. Children have become very accustomed to after school pit stops at the fast food chains, school lunch programs, pizza, hot dogs and French fries as their main staples. In fact, the goal of the school lunch programs is not to provide good nutrition to children but rather to make money for school administrators and the companies providing the meals.

Weight gain among American children begins in early childhood. During the first year of a child's life fat cells are developing. Feeding too much food during this time will lead to an increase in fat cell development. These additional fat cells do not go away. They stay forever. Only the size of the fat cells may change based on the amount of food consumed. Fat cells shrink when you eat less and increase when you eat more. Bottle-feeding stimulates babies to eat more, develop overeating habits and increases fat cell production. With bottle-feeding, babies set up the time of eating and feeding. Bottle-feeding tends to create isolation between mother and baby and contributes to a loss in the loving relationship between a mother and child. Breast milk has ingredients that protect the baby against infection, allergy, and digestive problems such as gas, constipation and stomach pain. Breast milk has less protein than cow's milk, which permits the baby to develop at a more natural rate. Breast milk also has fewer calories than cow's milk. More importantly, with breast-feeding the mother sets up the time and frequency of feeding. Therefore, breast-fed babies consume fewer calories, protein, and growth hormones than their bottle-fed counterparts. Also, their stomachs do not become enlarged, as is the case with most bottle-fed infants.

Since the 1960's bottle-feeding has become the traditional method of feeding infants in America. Only recently have some women returned to breast-feeding. Most mothers do not breast-feed because they are working full-time and leave the childcare to a grandparent, a babysitter or agency. Bottle-feeding causes many problems for the baby. Regular dairy milk contains very high protein, contributing to rapid weight gain and early maturation. In the natural life cycle of a calf, the cow's milk is formulated to promote rapid weight gain and growth. In the natural life cycle of a human baby, maturation (growth and development) takes place at a much slower rate because we live longer than cattle do. In addition, cows milk contains antibodies and steroids that can cause unnecessary digestive problems, infection and allergies to infants. It is also indicated that breast-fed babies tend to be more relaxed and happier than bottle-fed babies due to the mutual satisfaction derived from the closer relationship between mother and infant. Other studies report that breast-feeding may be a contributing factor in preventing breast cancer.

How to prevent childhood obesity

To deal successfully with combating childhood obesity, we must change our thinking and approach to what we feed our children starting at birth. The following changes have the greatest effect:

- Breast-feeding rater than bottle-feeding.

- When the infant is ready, introduce solid foods. Table foods that are finely chopped or puréed can be used rather than commercial can, jar or bottle foods that tend to be high in fat, salt, calories, and additives.

- Schools need to offer one hour a day of physical activity to children.

- Increase physical activity levels outside of school.

- Schools need to offer healthier food options such as salad, yogurt, sandwiches, and fresh fruit and remove pizza, hot dogs, chips and cookies.

- Families should prepare more meals at home and eat together.

PART II

HOW TO SELECT A PROPER DIET

2

WHERE DO WE GET OUR NUTRITIONAL KNOWLEDGE?

Based upon the misleading and often confusing information regarding nutrition and its effect on health, I have devoted a portion of this book to educate the public on basic nutrition. This section provides you with up to date information concerning the functions, sources, and requirements of good carbohydrates, fats, proteins, vitamins, and minerals. It also includes the daily requirements of water and the danger of excess water intake. I hope the information helps you with making good choices in the selection of your diet.

The rise in chronic diseases such as high cholesterol, high blood pressure, diabetes, heart disease, stroke, and cancer is very closely connected to poor nutrition and eating habits. Foods high in fat, sugar, salt, additives, and preservatives and overeating are responsible for this surge in chronic health problems. Unfortunately, drug companies take advantage of the situation by producing all kinds of medications to control but not cure these illnesses. Patients use these drugs day after day for many years without addressing the underlying root of the problem. It is a goldmine for the drug companies. Yet, each drug has its side effects and can sometimes cause more harm than benefit to the people taking them. The solution to our chronic health problems lies in proper selection of food, not drugs. In my clinic I have helped many people to lower their blood pressure, reduce blood sugar and cholesterol levels, and lower their body weight by planning a proper diet. I strongly believe that anyone can do it by himself or herself if they know how to choose proper foods. In this section my goal is to provide the best nutrition knowledge for you so that you will be able to plan your own diet, lose weight and improve your health.

Today in America, newspapers, television talk shows, and magazine articles are the principle sources of nutritional information for the general public. These sources have a strong influence on food trends and nutritional beliefs for millions of consumers. According to recent studies, the majority of available information does not have any scientific basis and is not reliable data. Media sources promote pills, herbs and drugs for losing weight and for curing a variety of diseases. Nutritional hustlers are cleaning up financially by stalking our fears and promising hopes with misleading information and credentials. They dominate television info-mercials and commercial publications. Television talk show hosts love these notions because they attract large audiences. The diet hustlers advise people who eat poorly, they do not have to worry, but just take their food supplement. They claim that natural vitamins are better than synthetic vitamins that brown eggs are better than white eggs, and that brown sugar is better than white sugar so that they can sell their products at high prices. In actuality, there is no difference between these products. White eggs are just as good as brown eggs. Synthetic vitamins have the same effect as natural vitamins. Another group claims they can identify a person's nutritional deficiencies by hair analysis. In fact, hair analysis after being studied has been found to be useless as a screening device to detect nutritional deficiency.

Television talk show hosts give a boost to the diet industry quacks when they ask what all these herbs do for you. They quickly reply that their products can improve vigor, vitality and memory, as well as fight against insomnia and cancer. Other quacks buy 30 minutes of television time to promote the power of enzymes. They claim that their enzyme products taken by mouth aid digestion and prevent acid reflux, constipation, and bloatedness. But in actuality, enzymes taken by mouth do not function like enzymes within the body. They preach about all the wonderful things our bodies can experience by taking their vitamins, minerals, herbs, and enzymes, and that harmful things happen to our bodies if we neglect to heed their advice. They conveniently neglect to inform listeners that a well balanced diet could provide all the nutrients your body needs. Health food quacks promote any number of unreliable supplements with all kinds of claims. Their claims are based upon faulty explanations of animal research. The most notorious of these product claims was tryptophan, an amino acid. For a long time it was marketed as a product for insomnia, depression and weight loss. Then in 1989, the use of this product caused a serious health hazard called eosinophelia mylgio syndrome, a rare disease characterized by swelling arms and legs, skin rash, fever, and joint pain. Not surprisingly the most widespread area of false information today is in the promotion of health foods and health food supplements. A large number of people are being misled regarding the need for these products. Health food industries use the vast and growing folklore surrounding nutrition, which is being built up by pseudoscientific literature in books, pamphlets, and magazines. As a result, millions of people are attempting self-medication for imaginary and real illnesses with a multitude of more or less irrational food items. Health food quackery today can only be compared to the patent medicine craze that reached its highest peak in the last century.

Present day nutrition scientists agree, that most chronic diseases, such as heart disease, cancer, diabetes, and digestive diseases are all rooted in the food we eat. Our diet can determine how we feel, look, and act. The food we eat can physiologically and psychologically affect our mood, our thinking, our energy, our self-confidence and our power of determination. In short, food can influence your zest for life and the fulfillment you derive from life. Physiologically, food affects our vigor, energy, and vitality, as well as our level of fatigue and exhaustion.

Food has the ability to determine how you feel, look, and act. It can influence whether you are grouchy or cheerful, whether you think clearly or confusedly, get pleasure from your work or make it drudgery. Our diet can also make the difference between a day ending with contentment, leading to a relaxing evening or ending with fatigue, forcing us to retire early. Most people talking about nutrition are food faddists or celebrities who have no scientific training. They peddle a tremendous amount of misinformation. The most important fact regarding good nutrition concerns not how much we eat, but what we eat. On average, foods are high in fat, salt, and chemical additives, which are responsible for most health problems we face, especially the problem of obesity. If we reduce the amount of fat, salt, and chemical additives in our diets and add some physical activity to our daily lives, we will be able to combat most of the major health problems, including obesity, as was done by generations before us.

Carbohydrates

Carbohydrate is the ideal energy source for most bodily functions. No food substances can provide a better fuel to the brain and nervous system than carbohydrates. The central nervous system is entirely dependent upon carbohydrates. Other food substances, such as protein, fat, and alcohol are not efficient fuels. If they are used in large amounts, they may produce very harmful effects. For example, a large amount of protein in the body increases uric acid and causes kidney problems. Over consumption of fat is responsible for heart disease and hardening of the blood vessels.

Carbohydrates have always been an important source of energy for people around the world. Lack of carbohydrate in the diet has been identified with causing tension, mental confusion, and poor reaction time. A person whose blood sugar falls below normal becomes progressively more irritable, grouchy, moody, depressed, and uncooperative. Since the brain can derive its energy only from carbohydrate foods; danger of blackout or fainting can occur if the supply falls below normal levels. On the other hand, if a diet provides adequate amounts of carbohydrates, blood sugar goes up and energy is easily produced, resulting in feeling better, feeling full of drive, and the ability to think quickly and clearly. Your attitude is composed and cheerful. Your disposition is at its best.

Classification of Carbohydrates

Carbohydrates are divided into two groups:

- Complex Carbohydrates

- Non-Complex Carbohydrates

This classification system is based on their effects on health.

Complex Carbohydrates

Complex carbohydrates occur in natural forms not altered by industrial processing. They are found in fruits, vegetables, rice, and potatoes to name a few. These carbohydrate foods have special characteristics:

- They are very high in vitamins, minerals, fiber, natural sugar, and natural water

- They are very low in salt, cholesterol, calories, and chemical additives

Non-Complex Carbohydrates

These foods are altered through industrial processing.
They are:

- Low in vitamins, minerals, and fiber

- High in fat, additives, salt, and calories

Complex carbohydrate foods such as corn, rice, potatoes, wheat bread, natural fruits, and vegetables can provide ample and nutritious fuel to the body and maintain your blood sugar within the normal range. These foods prevent blood sugar fluctuation, which is very important in the prevention of fatigue. Fruits and vegetables provide vitamins, minerals, and good sources of fiber. On the other hand, concentrated sugars and products made from them such as pastries, cakes, and soft drinks are absorbed rapidly into the blood circulation in a matter of minutes and raise the blood sugar very high. This rapid rise in blood sugar over stimulates the healthy pancreas to pour insulin into the blood. The insulin, in turn, causes the liver and muscles to withdraw sugar and store it as fat, thus preventing it from being lost in the urine. As the consumption of concentrated sugar continues, more sugar will pour into the blood, calling for the pancreas to send more insulin, and the pancreas obeys. The blood sugar drops below normal as a result of too much insulin. Then, a person begins to experience the symptoms of hypoglycemia, which can be fatigue, anxiety, stress, headache, sweating and/or dizziness. If the consumption of concentrated sugar products continues, the pancreas becomes fatigued and weakens. It no longer will produce an adequate amount of insulin to keep the blood sugar in the normal range. The blood sugar goes up and it cannot be controlled without medication. This is the beginning stage of diabetes.

Digestion of Carbohydrates

Before carbohydrates can produce energy, they must be converted into sufficiently small units to pass through the walls of the intestine into the bloodstream. The process by which complex carbohydrates such as pasta or rice are reduced to their component units is one aspect of digestion. An enzyme called amylase brings about virtually all the changes involved.

Amylase is present in two digestive juices:

• The saliva in the mouth

• The pancreatic juice in the small intestine

The salivary amylase mixes with the food in the mouth and converts it to simpler carbohydrates called dextrins. No digestion of carbohydrates takes place in the stomach because the stomach possesses no starch splitting enzyme. From the stomach, the digestive mass passes to the small intestine where pancreatic amylase attack complex carbohydrates and convert them into glucose and fructose, making them ready for absorption into the blood stream. From the intestinal wall, the simple sugars are carried to the liver. In the liver, part of glucose is converted into glycogen and stored in the liver and part of it is released into the bloodstream to be carried to various cells in the body. Most glucose will be utilized as an immediate source of energy for the cells. The nerve and lung cells depend entirely on glucose as a source of energy. The excessive sugar in the liver is converted into fat and then transported in the bloodstream to the adipose tissue cells.

Characteristics of Non-Complex Carbohydrates

These carbohydrates such as sugar, cake, and pastry are very high in salt, cholesterol, fat, calories, chemical additives, and sugar. They are very low in vitamins, minerals, and fiber. Examples of non-complex carbohydrates are cake, pie, potato chips, cookies, and muffins.

These foods are the underlying source for many human illnesses such as diabetes, constipation, and digestive disorders. In terms of chemical structure, carbohydrates are divided into three groups:

- Mono-Saccharides

- Di-Saccharides

- Poly-Saccharides

Mono-Saccharides

These carbohydrates are made up from three groups:

- Glucose

- Fructose

- Galactose

Glucose is found in fruits, vegetables, honey, and in the human blood.

Fructose is formed together with glucose in fruits.

The sweetness of the fruit is due to the amount of fructose it contains. Therefore, the higher the fructose, the sweeter the fruit.

Galactose is found only in mothers' milk. It is essential for infant nutrition.

Di-Saccharides

These carbohydrates are made up from two simple sugars.

These are divided into three groups:

- Lactose

- Sucrose

- Maltose

Lactose is found only in milk. Human milk has more lactose than cow's milk. Lactose is made up from glucose and galactose, and it is not very sweet.

Lactose Intolerance

Some people cannot digest milk. They lack an enzyme. In such circumstances, lactose passes into the large intestine where it is fermented by the intestinal bacteria, causing diarrhea, gas, and abdominal pain. People whose ancestors came from the Mediterranean areas around Italy, Greece, and North Africa tend to have a problem digesting milk. Italian, Spanish, Greek, Jewish, and Black heritage people are included in this group. The reason being that these nationalities consumed cheese rather than milk. For this reason they did not develop the digestive enzyme for milk, called "amylase," hence will not have tolerance for milk. For those who cannot tolerate milk, cheese should be used as a source of calcium. Cheese does not contain lactose. During the cheese making process, lactose is converted into lactic acid, which does not require amylase for proper digestion.

Sucrose

Sucrose is found in sugar cane, sugar beets, maple syrup, and fruits. Table sugar is made up from sucrose.

Poly-Saccharides

Poly-Saccharides are composed of glucose linked together to form very large molecules. Poly-Saccharides are divided into three groups, called starches, cellulose, and glycogen.

Starches occur in plants and plant seeds such as potatoes, wheat, rice, corn, and oats. Starches represent half the dietary carbohydrates. Each plant develops a starch characteristic of its species. The starch of potatoes can be distinguished from that of rice. Animals store a limited amount of carbohydrates. It is stored primarily in the liver and muscles. An adult human stores only about 340 grams of glycogen in the body. The capacity of the liver and muscles to store glycogen can be increased by manipulating the diet in association with exercise. This procedure is known as carbohydrate loading.

Cellulose is widely distributed among plants and is the only component of dietary fiber having a fibrous structure. The basic unit of cellulose is glucose. Humans cannot utilize cellulose as a source of energy because humans do not have any enzyme to digest cellulose. Animals such as cows and horses can utilize it for energy, but cellulose has a tremendous beneficial effect on human health. It protects the digestive system from cancer, constipation, and many other digestive problems, which are mentioned in the section devoted to The Effects of Fiber in Human Nutrition.

Glycogen. Foods have very little glycogen. Glycogen has been called animal starch and is manufactured in the liver and muscles from glucose. Glycogen serves as a source of stored energy, which the liver can easily break down into glucose when needed to maintain the blood sugar level or to use for energy. Most of the glycogen is stored in the muscles and in the liver. Glycogen plays a very important role in physical exercise and carbohydrate loading.

Foods High in Fiber

Complex Carbohydrates
GROUP A BREADS (Whole Wheat)

Rye Bread
Corn
Pasta
Potatoes
Rice

GROUP B FRUITS

Apples
Cantaloupe
Citrus Fruits
Grapes
Grapefruit
Honeydew

Pineapple
Pear
Plum
Watermelon
Peaches
Prunes
Dried Fruits

GROUP C VEGETABLES

Asparagus
Broccoli
Brussel Sprouts
Carrots
Cabbage
Cauliflower
Celery
Corn
Eggplant
Endive
Lettuce
Green Beans
Lima Beans
All other beans
Mushrooms
Okra
Peas (all types)
Radishes
Spinach
Squash
Sauerkraut
Tomatoes
Turnips
Watercress

GROUP D (CEREALS)

Oatmeal
Shredded Wheat
Bran Cereal

Puffed Rice
Raw, unprocessed bran

GROUP E BREADS

Whole Wheat
Cracked Wheat
Buckwheat
Corn Bread

NOTE:

You can eat any other vegetable or fruit that is not listed in this group provided they are not processed.

Foods Low in Fiber

GROUP A

White Rice
Cream of Wheat
Farina
White Bread
Pasta
Pastries
Pie
Cakes
Macaroni
Spaghetti
Noodles

Foods Without Fiber

GROUP B

Beef
Veal
Lamb
Fish
Shrimp

Lobster
Ham
Turkey
Tuna
Pork
Eggs
Margarine
Vegetable Oils
Ketchup
Chicken
Bacon
Butter
Cream
Salad Dressing
Corn Oil
Olive Oil
Ice Cream

3

FATS

Fats, such as butter, vegetables oils, lard, and margarine are familiar to everyone. The average American consumes about one-forth of a pound of fat (110 grams) per day, a practice not without its nutritional hazards. In Japan or China a very small percent (6%) of the diet comes from fat whereas Americans consume more than forty percent fat in their total calorie intake. Fat is an organic substance insoluble in water, but soluble in alcohol. The principle food sources contributing fat to the diet are butter, margarine, lard, and vegetable oils. Other sources include invisible fats found in cream, milk products, egg yolk, avocados, and nuts.

Classification of Fats

Fats are divided into two groups:

- Saturated Fats

- Unsaturated Fats

Saturated Fats:

This kind of fat comes from animal origins. They are solid at room temperature. Fats found in meat, butter, chicken and dairy products are saturated. These fats are major contributors to cardiovascular disease, cancer, high blood pressure, high cholesterol, and obesity.

Unsaturated Fats:

These fats come from plants, such as corn, olives, nuts, and vegetables and are in a liquid state. They are not harmful to the individual health, but excessive use of this fat will contribute to obesity. Each gram of fat produces nine calories no matter what its origin (animal or plant).

Functions of Fats:

Fats play a very important role in the human body. Without fat, the body cannot carry on its vital functions. These functions are:

- Production of energy

- Protection of the vital organs

- Production of hormones

- Insulation of the body

- Protection of the skin from radiation

- Absorption of Vitamins A, D, E, and K

Digestion of Fat

Fats are digested primarily in the small intestine. No digestion of fat takes place in the stomach. The function of the stomach in relation to fat digestion is to liquidize it. As fat enters the small intestine, the presence of fat stimulates the intestinal wall to secrete a hormone that is carried to the gall bladder by the blood. This hormone stimulates the contraction of the gall bladder, thereby forcing bile into the common duct and then into the small intestine.

Bile has several important functions:

- It stimulates peristalsis, which is a natural movement of the digestive tract to help move the bowel

- To neutralize an acid environment so as to provide the optimum condition for the digestion of fat

- To increase the effectiveness of enzyme action on fat digestion

Fatty food reduces the mobility of the digestive tract. Foods high in fat remain in the stomach longer than those that are low in fat. Fried foods are digested at a much slower rate. Lack of bile acid interferes with digestion of fat causing gas, bloatedness, and constipation.

Lack of bile acid is caused by:

- Gallstones blocking the common bile duct

- Infection of the common bile duct

Metabolism of Fats

Fat enters the cells and it is used in several ways:

- Some of the fats are oxidized and produce energy

- Others are stored in the cells

- Some others are used for the synthesis of hormones

- The remaining fat is stored in the adipose tissues and forms a layer known as subcutaneous fat

Consumption of fat in America

The predominant component in the American diet is fat. Some of these dietary fats are identified as visible fats and oils such as butter, margarine, solid fat, and fat surrounding meat. The other fats are called invisible fats including that fat marbled throughout meat fibers, in eggs, in milk, nuts, and legumes. Today, sixty percent of the dietary fat comes from animal sources and forty percent from vegetable sources. In 1910, fat consumption was approximately 125 grams per day, but by 1980, the consumption of fat increased to 168 grams per day. The consumption of fat in the American diet is much higher than other countries in the world. For instance, consumption of fat in Europe is 109 grams per day.

There is a very strong correlation between fat consumption and cardiovascular disease. As the consumption of fat increases, the instance of cardiovascular diseases, cancer, and obesity increases. To prevent disease and improve our health and well being, we must take the following into consideration:

- A reduction in the total fat calories from 45% to 25%

- A reduction of total fat from animal sources

- Remove visible fat from meat and poultry

- Use more fat from vegetable sources

- Increase the consumption of complex carbohydrates

- Avoid the consumption of fried foods

Why should we reduce our saturated fat intake?

Saturated fats in the diet will affect the level of serum cholesterol by changing the number of receptors to low-density cholesterol in the liver. When saturated fats are decreased in the diet, the numbers of high-density cholesterol receptors are increased in the liver. The liver is the major organ in the body for pulling and clearing low-density cholesterol from the bloodstream and sending it to the digestive system for excretion. Therefore our goal should be to reduce our total saturated fat consumption to not more than ten percent of total calorie intake.

Tips to reduce saturated fat in your diet

To reduce the amount of saturated fats in the diet, we must do the following:

- Steam, bake, or broil foods

- Use seasonings such as lemon, garlic, onion, and other non-salt spices to improve the taste

- Use corn and olive oils in place of animal fats

- Replace whole milk with skim or one percent milk

- Use plain, low-fat yogurt in place of sour cream

- Trim all visible fat from meat and poultry

- Remove all skin from poultry before cooking

- Use a non-stick pan for cooking so that there is no need to use fat

- Avoid high fat cheese

- Avoid using coconut oil, palm oil, butter, margarine, coffee creamer, ice cream, cream cheese, sausage, and fried foods

Cholesterol

Cholesterol occurs only in foods of animal origin. Liver, kidney, and eggs contain the largest amount of cholesterol among foods. Other sources of cholesterol in the diet are meats, shellfish, and dairy products. Cholesterol is a form of fat. The body can produce all that it needs and therefore is not dependent on dietary cholesterol.

Cholesterol plays many important roles in the body:

• It is a very important structural component of all cells in the body

• It is essential for normal development of the brain and nervous system

• Cholesterol is the important substance in the skin that makes it impervious to water

• The breakdown of cholesterol by the liver produces bile acid, without which digestion of fat cannot occur

• Cholesterol is a vital component of many hormones, including sex hormones

• Cholesterol in the skin, with help from the sun, produces Vitamin D. Vitamin D is essential for absorption of calcium in the digestive system

• Cholesterol also protects skin against radiation (skin cancer)

Dangers of high cholesterol

Blood cholesterol comes from two sources. The liver synthesizes most of the body's cholesterol, but some is obtained through the diet. Cholesterol has repeatedly shown to be associated with a high risk of coronary artery disease and myocardial infarction. Further research has drawn a distinction between high-density lipoprotein (HDL) and low-density lipoprotein (LDL). Now it is believed that the balance between HDL and LDL is more important than total cholesterol in the blood. The risk of coronary heart disease increases as LDL increases and HDL decreases. That is because HDL promotes the removal of excess cholesterol from the cells and its excretion from the body. In contrast, LDL picks up the cholesterol from ingested fats and from cells that synthesize it in the body and delivers it to the blood vessels. The concentration of cholesterol in the cells within the lining of the arteries contributes to the build up of arteriosclerotic plaques. Experts agree that we must keep our blood cholesterol in the normal range. No one should have cholesterol above 200, especially those who are overweight and those who have a family history of heart disease. The ratio of HDL and LDL must be kept low. You must keep the high-density cholesterol above 50 mg and your low-density cholesterol under 130 mg. Low-density blood cholesterol is the major cause of heart disease. It is vitally important that we should lower the LDL cholesterol. Numerous studies have suggested that several factors play a vital role in the reduction of LDL. Among them are:

- Decrease dietary cholesterol

- Decrease calories from saturated fat

- Decrease calories from fat

- Increase fiber in your diet (fruits, vegetables, whole grain products)

- Reduce body weight

- Participate in aerobic exercise

Dietary fat is also associated with the second leading cause of death in the United States, which is cancer. A diet high in fat is a major factor in the development of breast, colon, rectal, and prostrate cancers. Four major diseases are also associated with high intake of animal fat and a high percentage of other body fat. These diseases are:

- Obesity

- Cardiovascular disease

- Diabetes

- Cancer

Cardiovascular Disease

Cardiovascular disease is a disorder of the heart and blood vessels. These diseases include heart attack, stroke, high blood pressure, and atherosclerosis. These diseases are responsible for one out of every two deaths in America.
The major risk factors are:

- High blood cholesterol

- Consumption of high dietary animal fats

How to increase high-density cholesterol

- Increase the consumption of fish, especially bluefish and salmon

- Increase fruits and vegetables in the diet

- Increase whole grain products

- Increase the level of physical activities

- Avoid consumption of beef, pork, and lamb, whole milk dairy products, such as cheese, butter and margarine, salad dressing and canned sauces

Essential fatty acid

One of the most important reasons to include fat in the diet is to supply linoleic acid. Linoleic acid is an essential fatty acid and must be obtained from foods because the body is unable to synthesize it. Lack of this substance will produce certain symptoms.
Among them are:

- Dry skin

- Dermatitis

- Damage to the hair follicle

- Growth retardation

Sources of Linoleic Acid:

- Corn oil

- Sunflower oil

- Soybean oil

   To obtain a sufficient amount of linoleic acid, corn oil should be used for cooking. That is the reason I have included corn oil in my recipes. Fat is a very important substance and it has many vital functions in the body. Lack of fat in the diet causes many abnormalities. Most importantly is the type of fat in the diet. Some fat is used as part of the structure of every cell. The brain, nerves, and skin need certain types of fats called essential fatty acids. Hormones and sex glands are made up of essential fatty acids, which are linoleic acid, linolenic acid, and arachidonic acid. Lack of these acids in the diet cause the hair to become dry and thin and the skin to become thick and scaly, especially the skin on the face. Eczema may develop. By adding these essential fatty acids to the diet, the skin clears up and eczema disappears.

A certain amount of fat is used by the body to stimulate the production of bile acid, which is essential for the digestion of fat. Low levels of bile acid causes abnormal digestion of fat, producing stomach gas, bloatedness, and constipation. Abnormal fat digestion also prevents absorption of Vitamins A, D, and K. Sources of essential fatty acids are corn oil, vegetable oil, soybean, and cottonseed oil. Very little essential fatty acids are found in animal fats.

4

PROTEINS

Protein gets it's name from a Greek word meaning "of first importance." Proteins are the key components of all living organisms and are essential constituents of blood and the nucleus of every cell. Twenty percent of body weight is composed of protein. Without protein, life cannot be sustained.

Protein is made up from carbon, oxygen, hydrogen, and nitrogen. The basic units of protein are amino acids. When protein is digested in the body, it becomes an amino acid and it is the amino acid that enters the blood stream. There are 22 amino acids that the body needs to perform its major functions. Eight of these amino acids are essential and must be provided from the outside because the body cannot make them.

Classification of protein

From a nutritional point of view, proteins are divided into two groups.
They are:

- Essential proteins

- Nonessential proteins

Essential Proteins:

This type of protein comes from animal sources such as seafood, beef, lamb, pork, eggs, and dairy products. Without essential protein, growth and the maintenance of the body will be impaired and the body will not have the capacity to fight infections. The adult body needs 80 to 100 grams of essential protein per day. Pregnant women, children and people who are under emotional stress need more protein.

Sources of Essential Proteins:

All essential proteins come from animal sources. No essential proteins can be found in plant foods. Good sources of protein are:

Chicken	Turkey	Dairy Products
Eggs	Meat (lamb, pork, beef)	Fish (all types)
Shellfish		

Nonessential Proteins:

These types of proteins come from plant sources, such as corn, bread, rice, fruits, legumes, and potatoes. Protein from plants cannot provide adequate amounts of essential protein to meet the requirements for growth and maintenance of the body. These proteins must be supplemented by animal protein. Combinations of essential protein and nonessential protein will provide all the nutrients that the body needs for growth and development of muscle tissue as well as for bone, blood, and antibodies.

Sources of Nonessential Proteins:

Wheat	Corn	Rice
Pasta	Potatoes	Beans
Fruits	Vegetables	

To maintain our bodies in good health, we need a high quality protein. Meat, fish, fowl, milk, cheese, yogurt, and eggs are superior sources of high quality proteins. Proteins are made up from amino acids containing nitrogen, which are lacking in other food sources. Not only does the protein of milk differ from those of cereals, but also the protein in all parts of our body varies due to the different combinations of amino acids that form them. When these proteins are eaten, the digestive process of a healthy person breaks them down into amino acids that pass into the blood and are then carried throughout the body. The cells select the amino acids they need, using them to construct new body tissue and for such vital substances as antibodies, hormones, enzymes, and blood cells. Every second our body's protein is being broken down by enzymes in our cells, and if our health is to be maintained, then amino acids must be available for immediate replacement.

When our diet has more protein available than our body needs, the liver withdraws amino acids from the blood and changes them into storage proteins. These excessive proteins will be converted into glucose and fat by the liver, and the nitrogen of the protein will be excreted in the urine. The glucose and fat will be used for energy or will be stored as fat. Some of these essential amino acids are used for treatment of diseases.

The eight essential amino acids are:

Methionine	Phenylalanine	Threonine	Valine
Leucine	Isoleucine	Tryptophan	Lysine

Two other amino acids are essential for growth. During childhood the diet must supply them. They are histidine and arginine. The value of any protein depends on the number and amount of essential amino acids it contains. Proteins containing the eight essential amino acids in generous amounts are called complete. If enough of any complete protein such as milk is consumed, it alone can support health. A protein lacking one or more essential amino acid or supplying too little of an essential amino acid to support life is an incomplete protein. Protein from meat, fish, eggs, milk, steak, cheese, and other animal sources have higher values for health than protein from vegetables, cereals, breads, potatoes, and pasta.

Extensive research has been done with both animals and humans to find the specific symptoms of ill health that occur when certain amino acids are lacking. For example, when the diet of animals or babies lack tryptophan, methionine or isoleucine, the liver cannot produce the blood proteins albumin and globulin (antibodies), therefore urine can no longer be collected normally. Swelling known as edema and susceptibility to infection can result. Methionine has been found to be particularly deficient in the diet of children with chronic rheumatic fever and of women suffering from the toxemia of pregnancy. In animals, including humans, a lack of tryptophan or methionine causes the hair to fall out. Lack of phenylalanine causes the eyes to become blood shot or cataracts to form.

Functions of Proteins

Proteins provide a key life force. They are crucial to the minute-by-minute regulation and maintenance of the various functions of our bodies. Vital body functions such as blood clotting, fluid balance, hormone and enzyme production, and cell repair all require protein. Our bodies are largely made up from protein, including skin, hair, nails, bones, muscles, brain, and all internal organs. Only when high quality protein is supplied can each cell act normally and keep itself in constant repair. When we receive an inadequate amount of good quality protein, cells lose their elasticity, strength, and energy.

Protein builds and repairs tissues:

Lack of protein causes the cells, tissues, muscles, and bones to become weak. The heart cannot push the blood through the blood vessels and the lungs cannot bring in fresh air, causing the blood pressure to go up. Because of this, fewer nutrients can be delivered to the tissues, resulting in fatigue, lack of energy, and emotional stress. Another cause of fatigue, which is common, is anemia or lack of red blood cells, which are made up almost entirely from protein. Red blood cells carry oxygen to the cells where the oxygen combines with food to produce energy. Low levels of red cells in the blood circulation are an indication of anemia or lack of energy.

Protein prevents infection:

Adequate protein is needed to produce various white blood cells. These white cells in the blood help to protect the body from invasion of pathogens. They are the armed forces of the body that guard us twenty-four hours a day. Some of these cells circulate in the blood and in the lymph system. Others are stationed in the walls of blood vessels, in the air sacs of the lungs, and in other tissues. When bacteria invade the body, these cells attack and destroy them right away. When the number of these cells decline, the body loses its immunity and becomes infected.

Protein maintains water balance:

Protein in the blood is responsible for maintaining the water level in the body. Pressure inside arteries pushes the blood into the capillaries and then into the tissues in order to supply nutrients to these tissues. The pressure produced by protein in the blood attracts the fluid back into the blood stream, thus controlling fluid balance in the circulation. Whenever the level of protein supply becomes inadequate, edema results. Edema leads to many serious medical problems; among them are heart damage, high blood pressure, respiratory problems, and joint pain. It also causes fatigue, anxiety, and lack of sleep.

Proteins build enzymes:

Enzymes produce all our energy in the body. Enzymes are organic substances whose principle component is protein. Enzymes are necessary for digestion of foods in the digestive system. Enzymes break down foods into small particles that can be dissolved in water and passed into the circulation. The stomach, small intestine, and pancreas can only produce enzymes when the supply of protein is adequate. The stomach walls, as well as the intestine and colon walls, must be kept strong in order to have a good digestive process.

How to select good protein:

As it was discussed previously, protein plays a very important role in growth and maintenance of the body. However, the type of protein the diet is a crucial factor we must be concerned with. Protein from certain sources contains not only saturated fat, but also growth hormones that are responsible for various cancers in man. The protein of lamb, beef, and pork contain a lot of saturated fats and growth hormones. Proteins from these animal sources should be reduced in the diet as much as possible.

Problems associated with these animals are:

• They store fat not only in between the muscle and skin, but also inside the muscle itself. That is the reason no matter what you do, you still will get a lot of saturated fat from these sources.

• Growth hormones are injected into these animals for two reasons: (1) to increase body mass and (2) so that farmers can shorten the length of maturation of these animals. It is a very profitable method for cattle ranchers but dangerous for consumers.

In order to obtain good protein, we must consume our protein from the following sources:

Chicken	Turkey	Seafood
Legumes	Whole grains	Low fat dairy products

Who should increase protein intake

There are special groups of people who must consume more protein in their diets.

They are:

- Pregnant women who must support the growth of the fetus

- People who have undergone surgery

- People who are under stress

- People engaged in vigorous physical activities

- Children in the process of growth

Digestion of Protein

Inside the mouth, nothing happens to protein except that it is crushed and mixed with saliva. When protein reaches the stomach, it faces a very strong acid, which helps to denature or split the protein so that the stomach enzymes can attack it and break it down into small pieces. Even though the stomach walls are made up of protein, the stomach acid and enzymes do not attack these proteins because they are the only proteins in the body designed to resist strong acid. A coat of mucus, secreted by the stomach cells, protects the stomach wall. By the time the denatured protein arrives in the intestine, it is broken down into smaller pieces. In the small intestine the acid delivered by the stomach is neutralized by alkaline juice from the pancreas, making it possible for intestinal enzymes to accomplish the final breakdown of the protein. Digestion continues until almost all proteins are broken down into amino acids.

Absorption of Protein

Absorption of protein takes place all along the small intestine. The cells of the small intestine capture the amino acids and then release them into the bloodstream. Once they are circulating in the bloodstream, the amino acids are available to be taken up by any cell in the body. The cells can then make protein, either for their own use or for secretion into the lymph or blood systems for other uses such as enzymes, hormones, or antibodies. The breakdown of protein foods in the stomach is accomplished by pepsin and in the small intestine it is carried out by tripsin.

The best way to obtain proper protein

For optimal growth and well-being, the human body requires a combination of essential (animal) and nonessential (plant) protein. We cannot carry on the vital physiological activities of life without animal protein. Therefore a daily diet must contain some animal products, perhaps at about four ounces of animal protein per day. The rest may come from plant protein. When we combine animal protein with plant protein in the diet, both proteins become essential protein. A good example of this food combination is:

- Cheese sandwich

- Turkey sandwich

- Chicken with rice

- Beef with potatoes

- Salad with turkey

- Salad with cheese

- Pasta with cheese

- Seafood with rice

- Tuna sandwich

- Varieties of legumes with chicken, fish, turkey, beef or dairy products

- Yogurt with fruit

- Chicken soup

- Egg sandwich

- Cereal with milk

Such diets will promote both growth and maintenance of the body not only during growth periods, but also during adult life. It should be stressed that consuming large amounts of animal protein not only increases your risk of cardiovascular disease, but it also elevates the level of uric acid in the blood. A higher level of uric acid in the blood is responsible for gout. In addition, a higher uric acid level disturbs the normal range of pH of the blood. When the pH level of blood is disturbed, it will affect all physiological functions of the vital organs.

Vegetarians

For many countries over the world, a vegetarian diet is used as an alternative diet by a large number of people. But since 1970, especially in the Western world, many young people most of whom come from middle and upper middle class backgrounds turned to vegetarian foods for a variety of reasons. For some people it represents a form of religion or spiritual release through which they hope to purify their bodies and find a place in heaven or an "eternal world." For another group, the vegetarian diet represents a form of rejection of many aspects of affluent society. The vegetarian diet serves as a healer for other people. They believe that foods can replace medicine. They use vegetarian foods to heal diseases and illness. Still there are people who use a vegetarian diet to slow down the aging process and eventually find the fountain of youth.

Vegetarians Are Divided into Four Groups

True Vegetarian

This group believes that all life is sacred, and that no life should be destroyed. They do not consume any animal products or by products. An example would be religious sects in India. True vegetarians are likely to suffer serious nutritional problems such as:

- Vitamin deficiencies of Vitamins A, E, D, K, and Vitamin B12

- Mineral deficiencies of Iron, Calcium, Potassium, and Zinc

- Lack of energy

Energy supplied by vegetarian foods is not sufficient to provide an ample amount of energy to perform physical activities.

Lacto-Vegetarian

This group consumes all vegetable foods plus dairy products such as yogurt, cheese, milk, and butter. They avoid animal foods such as meat, poultry, seafood, and eggs.

Lacto-Ovo Vegetarian

This group avoids all animal products except eggs and dairy products. They consume, eggs, cheese, butter, yogurt, milk, and buttermilk, plus all vegetarian foods, such as fruits, vegetables, legumes, and whole grain products.

Quasi-Vegetarian

This group avoids all animal products except fish and seafood. They do not consume eggs or dairy products.

5

VITAMINS

History of Vitamins

The history of vitamins, their discovery and effects on deficiency diseases, is very fascinating. Vitamin investigation began with the search for dietary factors that would prevent or cure deficiency diseases such as scurvy, rickets, pellagra, night blindness, and hemorrhagic disease of newborns, to name a few. Although history cites evidence that the benefit of food ingredients (spices, herbs, etc.) dates back several hundred years, scientific knowledge of vitamins dates back only to the close of the nineteenth century.

In 1897 Christian Elgkman, described a disease in chickens resembling beriberi in man. He induced this disease by feeding milled rice to chickens. He discovered that feeding rice polishings could cure the symptoms. The polishings contained thiamine that prevented disease. This recognition of the importance of other factors besides carbohydrates, fats, and proteins in promoting health stimulated investigations by other workers, which led to the modern concept of vitamins. The young biologist, Dr. Casimer Funk, who in 1912, at the age of 28, coined the word "vitamin" meaning essential, promoted research in the field of vitamins. In 1914, he wrote the first book on vitamins. He proposed that the dietary deficiency diseases of beriberi, scurvy, pellagra, and rickets were caused by a lack in the diet of special substances, which we called vitamins. By 1920, vitamins were classified either as fat and water soluble, a distinction accepted by the scientific community.

What is a vitamin?

A vitamin is an organic compound other than protein, fat, or carbohydrate. Vitamins are essential for growth, production of energy, and maintenance of good health. Animals fed on pure fat, protein, carbohydrate, water, and minerals failed to grow because they lacked vitamins. Most foods contain a good supply of vitamins, but today foods are processed and do not contain adequate amounts of vitamins, therefore most people lack sufficient vitamins.

Characteristics of vitamins

- Vitamins are not food therefore they cannot satisfy hunger

- The human body cannot produce vitamins. They must come from outside sources, with exception to vitamin D.

- Each vitamin has a specific function in the body

- Some vitamins are fat-soluble and others are water-soluble, therefore they must be taken with food

- Coffee or alcohol work against vitamins, therefore they must not be used together

Important facts you should know about vitamins

A vitamin is defined as a coenzyme, an indispensable and essential, non-caloric, organic nutrient needed in tiny amounts in the daily diet. Coenzymes help other enzymes break down, absorb, and metabolize food. The role of the vitamin is to serve as a helper to cell metabolism, making it possible for nutrients to be digested, absorbed, metabolized, and/or built into new body structure. Vitamins are not oxidized themselves, but they help to liberate energy from food for human use.

Today, more than 90 million adult Americans take vitamin supplements. Some of these people are taking extremely large doses in the belief that the more vitamins you take, the more protection you get from disease. Each year increasing numbers of people report to hospitals for vitamin poisoning. Some vitamins are extremely harmful. Large doses of some vitamins may damage the liver and kidneys. One should know that the human body needs very tiny amounts of vitamins to carry on its physiological processes. Daily consumption of fruits and vegetables can meet vitamin requirements. Since most people eat very few fruits and vegetables, they may need to take vitamin supplements; however, we must be very careful not to overdose.

There is no difference between natural and synthetic vitamins. A cell picking up vitamins from the blood stream cannot tell the difference between vitamins derived from pills or from foods. Those who take vitamin supplements should take into consideration the following:

- Never take vitamins without food. You gain no benefit. Vitamins only aid digestion, absorption, and metabolism of foods; that is all.

- Coffee, tea and alcohol have an anti-vitamin effect. If vitamins are consumed with any of these beverages they lose their beneficial effect.

- Vitamins cannot satisfy hunger nor can they produce hunger

- There is no difference between synthetic vitamins and natural vitamins

- The intake of large dosages of vitamins is dangerous and can poison your body

Vitamin supplements

I hope that you have read and learned a great deal about nutrition education from the information that I have provided in this section. Now you know more than the average person about vitamins, minerals, protein, fat, carbohydrates and their roles in health promotion. Therefore, you can make food selections more wisely. Since the foods we consume today are not 100 percent natural, we may need certain vitamin or mineral supplements. On that basis, I recommend taking some vitamin and mineral supplements to meet the needs of the body.

There are two groups of vitamins, which are very important.

Group A—The antioxidant vitamins

They include Vitamin A, Vitamin C, and Vitamin E.
These vitamins are beneficial because:

- They protect the immune system and prevent infection

- They prevent cancer and protect the tissue from damage caused by free radicals

- They slow down the aging process

Recommended Supplements:

Vitamin A	10,000 I.U.
Vitamin C	500 Mg

Group B—These vitamins are involved in the production of energy.

They include Folic Acid, Vitamin B1, and Vitamin B12.
Recommended Supplements:

Folic Acid	400 Mcg
Vitamin B1	50 Mg
Vitamin B12	50 Mg

In addition to vitamins, there are certain minerals that are essential for the normal functions of the body. They include:

- Calcium—for the bones and muscles

- Zinc—for hair, skin, and protection against prostrate cancer

- Chromium—for production of energy

- Potassium—for prevention of water retention

Recommended Supplements:

Calcium	800 Mg
Chromium	200 Mg
Zinc	20 Mg
Potassium	100 Mg

Classification of Vitamins

Fat-soluble vitamins are only soluble in fat. They can be stored in the body. There is no need for daily intake. Excessive intake of these vitamins can be toxic and harmful and may cause liver damage.

The fat-soluble vitamins:

- Vitamin A   (Retinal)
- Vitamin D   (Calciferol)

- Vitamin E   (Tocopherol)
- Vitamin K

The water-soluble vitamins:

- Vitamin B1   (Thiamine)
- Vitamin B2   (Riboflavin)
- Niacin   (Nicotinic acid)
- Vitamin B6   (Pyridoxine)
- Folic Acid
- Pantothenic Acid
- Biotin
- Vitamin B12 (Cobalamin)
- Vitamin C

Vitamin A

Vitamin A was the first fat-soluble vitamin to be recognized. Two groups of research workers, McLean and Davis at the University of Wisconsin, and Mandel at Yale University made the discovery in 1913. They found that young animals became unhealthy and failed to grow on diets lacking natural fats. They also found that eyes become inflamed and infected but could be quickly relieved by the addition of a natural fat to their diets.

Functions

Vision—both day and night vision requires Vitamin A. But night vision depends on the Vitamin A mechanism entirely. A deficiency in Vitamin A causes difficulty seeing in the dark. When there is Vitamin A deficiency, you cannot see the road after your eyes have been exposed to the headlights of an oncoming car.

Itching and Burning Eyes—lack of Vitamin A may cause burning and itching eyes. Eyelids become inflamed and eyeballs become painful.

Skin—deficiency of Vitamin A affects the skin. The cells in the lower layer of the skin die and slough off. They plug oil sacs and pores, preventing oil from reaching the surface. The skin becomes so dry and rough that the entire body begins to itch. The roughness of the skin usually occurs first on the elbows, knees, buttocks, and the backs of the upper arms.

Mucous Membranes—protect the inside of the throat, nose, sinuses, middle ears, lungs, urinary tract, and the gall bladder from infection. If the diet is adequate in Vitamin A, the mucous membrane continuously protects the body. The role of a mucous membrane is to secrete mucous to cover the cells, preventing bacteria from reaching them. Bacteria cannot function in the mucous environment. They die.

Growth and Bone Development—Vitamin A is essential to the development of bone and teeth enamel. Lack of Vitamin A slows growth and development.

Immunity—Vitamin A deficiency increases susceptibility to bacterial, viral, or parasitic infections. It is because of this observation and the fact that Vitamin A is important in maintaining the integrity of the mucous membrane that Vitamin A is known as the anti-infection vitamin. Without Vitamin A the barrier system against infection is gone.

Anti-Cancer—several studies indicated that Vitamin A has a role in promoting normal functions of the epithelial cells and by doing so helps prevent the development of malignancy in these cells. For this reason, Vitamin A is being used in humans to treat cancer, especially the cancers of the skin, lungs, breast, and bladder.

Sources

The leading dietary sources of Vitamin A are liver, eggs, whole milk, butter, and cheese. Sources among vegetables are dark green, leafy and yellow vegetables such as collard, spinach, carrots, squash, and sweet potatoes. Fruit sources include peaches, cantaloupe, and other melons.

Requirements

The requirement of Vitamin A for men is 5000 I.U. per day. For women it is 4000 I.U. per day, but during pregnancy and lactation, the requirement increases to 6000 I.U. per day.

VITAMIN E

Evans and Bishop discovered Vitamin E in 1922 when they found that rats reared on a basic diet failed to reproduce until they were given a substance isolated from vegetable oil. After being given this substance, the rats produced robust offspring. This substance was given the name of Vitamin E or anti-sterility vitamin. In 1936, it was chemically identified.

Functions

Antioxidant—Vitamin E acts as an antioxidant. It serves to prevent unsaturated fatty acid from being destroyed in the body by oxygen. It also protects fatty-like substances such as sex hormones and adrenal hormones from destruction.

Prevents free radicals—from damaging the cell membrane. Free radicals speed up the aging process in humans. Vitamin E, by destroying free radicals, slows down the aging process.

Prevents anemia—many red blood cells die everyday. To replace the dying cells, the body needs Vitamin E. Vitamin E is very important during pregnancy. Deficiency in pregnant women causes anemia in the newborn baby. During space flights, astronauts who spent more than eight days in space lost between 20 to 30 percent of their red blood cells. When they returned to earth, they were extremely tired and their hearts so weakened that it puzzled their physicians. The reason discovered for these problems was due to the oxygen rich atmosphere, which rapidly destroyed unsaturated fatty acid in the cells.

Prevents blood clots—Vitamin E prevents the formation of a brown pigment produced by oxidation of unsaturated fatty acid by the presence of oxygen. These pigments prevent the production of an enzyme that dissolves the blood clot. This is the major problem in stroke, heart attack, phlebitis, and varicose veins.

Hemolytic anemia—newborn babies deficient in Vitamin E are prone to developing hemolytic anemia. This may be due to the feeding of formulas high in unsaturated fatty acids and iron. Formulas have a deficiency in Vitamin E, whereas human milk contains sufficient amounts to meet infant requirements. The major problem related to Vitamin E deficiency is muscle weakness; especially calf muscles become very painful during walking.

Sources

Vitamin E is found in the following foods: nuts, liver, eggs, wheat breads, vegetable oils, and green vegetables. Wheat germ oil is the richest source.

Requirements

The allowance for infants is 200 I.U. per day. For adult males and females it is 400 I.U. per day. A diet high in polyunsaturated fat such as vegetable oils requires more Vitamin E.

ANTIOXIDANTS

More than a million Americans are diagnosed with cancer each year. In an effort to avoid cancer, people should eat more fiber and reduce the consumption of meat and fats. In recent years scientists have realized that fruits and vegetables are the best defense against cancer. Today, the hidden world of natural chemicals in edible plants is unfolding. An explosion of compelling and consistent data associates diets rich in fruits and vegetables with lower cancer risk. Data from 23 epidemiological studies clearly shows that a diet rich in fruits and vegetables slashed colon cancer by 40%. Another study shows that women who ate few fruits and vegetables had 25% higher breast cancer than women who consumed more fruits and vegetables. Such evidence has encouraged scientists to try to analyze just what it is about fruits and vegetables that enable a diet rich in them to reduce cancer. They believe that it is not vitamins and minerals or proteins that are protecting the body from cancer, but biochemical substances called phytochemicals.

When life began, plants were anaerobic. They lived in a world without oxygen. As they evolved, they began to turn carbon dioxide into oxygen. They gradually polluted their own environment. In order to survive, plants were forced to develop chemicals (antioxidants) to defend against the unstable form of oxygen. These chemicals are called phytochemicals, many of which are brightly colored and give plants their vivid colors. These colors are key parts of an antioxidant defense system. In addition to resisting oxidation, these substances fight against viral attack, harsh weather, and other environmental forces. There are hundreds of phytochemicals, classified into several groups by chemical names, by primary food sources, and by anti-cancer action. Foods may contain numerous phytochemicals, each acting through one or more mechanisms.

Flavonoids

These chemicals are found in many fruits and vegetables. They reduce cancer risk by acting as antioxidants, blocking the action of carcinogens to cells by suppressing malignant changes in cells. They also interfere with the binding of hormones to cells, thus inhibiting cancer development.

Vitamin K

Vitamin K was discovered in 1935. Chickens fed on a ration seemingly adequate in all dietary essentials produced still experienced a severe hemorrhagic disease.

When chickens were additionally given hog liver, normal clotting time was restored. The hemorrhage was due to a lack of prothrombin, a compound required for a normal clotting of blood. This compound was called Vitamin K "Koagulation Vitamin."

Function

Vitamin K has one major function. It is necessary for normal clotting of blood. A deficiency of Vitamin K causes slow clotting time. Administering Vitamin K to mothers prior to the birth of the fetus has reduced the incidence of hemorrhage among newborns. A deficiency of Vitamin K may occur when diets lack green vegetables. Using too much antibiotic medicine inhibits the growth of intestinal microorganisms

Sources

There are two major sources of Vitamin K.

• Ingested foods

• Intestinal synthesis

Foods such as green vegetables, spinach, kale, broccoli, cabbage, lettuce, and alfalfa are the richest sources of Vitamin K. Vitamin K is also found in tomatoes, liver, soybeans, and eggs. Bacteria in the intestinal tract produce Vitamin K, but excessive use of antibiotic medicine destroys these beneficial bacteria and produces Vitamin K deficiency.

Requirement

No specific estimate of Vitamin K requirement has been made for humans, but 2 mg. of Vitamin K per day will correct Vitamin K deficiency in most cases. The suggested intake for adults is 70 mg. per day.

VITAMIN D

Vitamin D was discovered in 1930 and was first synthesized in 1936. The special role of this vitamin is to be sure that sufficient calcium, important to bone structure, is available in the blood. It is also very important in the maintenance of the normal serum level of calcium and phosphorus. The most obvious sign of Vitamin D deficiency is the abnormality of bones. Examples are rickets and osteoporosic conditions in which calcium, when withdrawn from bones, causes the bones to lose their minerals and become porous, weak, and easy to break. Some deafness can also be caused by Vitamin D deficiency, because sound is transmitted along tiny ear bones to the brain. These bones also degenerate due to Vitamin D deficiency. Prolonged breast-feeding without the mother taking Vitamin D supplements or omission of milk from the diet of children can lead to rickets. Earlier in the century, when there were no labor laws to govern child labor, a large number of children worked in factories for long hours and did not receive any sunlight. The disease of rickets was prevalent among these children. Rickets is a disease in which bones, especially the bones of the legs, are not calcified completely, and are unable to support the weight of the body. As a result, the bones become bent, resembling a bow. For that reason it is called bowlegs.

Requirement

The daily requirement of Vitamin D is not necessary because the excesses are stored in the body. Vitamin D is extremely toxic. Special care must be taken in regard to the usage of this supplement. The toxicity symptoms are headache, diarrhea, and nausea.

Sources

The major sources of Vitamin D are egg yolks, liver, butter, and fish oils. In the United States milk is fortified with Vitamin D, therefore milk can be a good source of this vitamin. The human body also makes Vitamin D when it is exposed to the sun. The sunlight converts the cholesterol contained in the skin into Vitamin D.

THE WATER SOLUBLE VITAMINS
THIAMINE

Thiamine is a water-soluble vitamin and cannot be stored in the body. It requires daily intake. Thiamine in the body acts as a coenzyme. It releases energy from carbohydrates and traps energy. Cells can utilize that energy when they perform work necessary for the body as a whole. Thiamine itself is not a source of energy, but it helps in the process of activating energy in food. This vitamin also plays an important role in the transmission of nerve impulses and in making the cardiac muscle efficient. A deficiency in Thiamine causes nausea, severe fatigue, loss of appetite, abnormal heartbeat, headache, insomnia, pain in the calf muscles, and numbness in the feet, confusion, short attention span, and depression.

Requirement

Since Thiamine cannot be stored in the body, it requires daily intake. Food containing Thiamine should be consumed on a daily basis. The requirement for adults is 2 mg. per day, but excessive alcohol intake increases the need for more of this vitamin.

Sources

Lean pork, liver, yeast, legumes, and fresh green vegetables are the major sources of this vitamin.

RIBOFLAVIN

Riboflavin is a coenzyme playing a vital role in the production of energy. It repairs damaged tissues and plays a role in the rate of growth. It also breaks down amino acids and fatty acids. A deficiency of this vitamin causes skin inflammation over the nose and eyes, failure to grow, and cracks on the lips corners of the mouth.

Requirements

The daily requirement for adults is 2 mg. per day, but children who are in the process of growth need more of this vitamin, at least 4 mg. per day.

Sources

Milk and milk products are the major sources of this vitamin. They provide half of the daily requirement. The other sources are dark green vegetables, nuts, seeds, and organ meats.

NIACIN

Niacin is necessary for energy production. It was discovered in 1867 and its importance was not found until much later when the disease called pellagra was discovered. Pellagra is a skin disease caused by lack of Niacin in the diet. This disease sometimes was called rough skin disease and occurred predominantly in the poor areas of Europe and in American South. After several years of research, the cause of the disease was a diet consisting of corn meal, pork fat, and molasses. The key nutrient that was lacking in the diet of pellagra patients was an amino acid called tryptophan, which is found in lean meats. Pellagra is characterized by a disturbance of every tissue. Symptoms include weakness of the muscles, loss of appetite, diarrhea, and a skin rash appearing on parts of the body exposed to the sun, confusion, and memory loss. Other symptoms include weakness, fatigue, and loss of appetite, indigestion, inflammation of the tongue, mouth, and the digestive tract. Anemia and vomiting may occur after a few months of Niacin deficiency. If the deficiency continues, memory loss, dizziness, and confusion develop.

VITAMIN B-6

Vitamin B6 or Pyridoxine is a water-soluble vitamin. It cannot be stored in the body and it must be taken on a daily basis either by eating foods that contain this vitamin or by taking supplements. The vitamin was discovered in 1926. Vitamin B6 plays a vital role in the formation of serotonin that controls the neurological activities of the brain. As a coenzyme, it converts tryptophan to Niacin. It also helps in the synthesizing of red blood cells.

Blood glucose levels are regulated by Vitamin B6. Lack of B-6 is associated with depression, nervous irritation, impaired immune system, severe fatigue, skin disorders, and water retention. Lack of Vitamin B6 interferes with the production of serotonin and amino butyric acid. Both these regulatory compounds control neurological conditions. Lack of B-6 increases irritability and if sustained may progress to seizures. Vitamin B6 deficiency can cause anemia characterized by fatigue, lack of energy, water retention, and disturbance of sleeping patterns.

Requirement

The daily requirement for adult men and women is 2 mg. per day. High intake of this vitamin may cause numbness of hands and feet.

Sources

The major sources of this vitamin are green leafy vegetables, fruits, fish, and meats.

FOLIC ACID

Folic acid is an anti-anemia vitamin and it is necessary for the production of red blood cells. It is responsible for the production of red blood cells and for their maturation as well. Without folic acid, red cells cannot develop into functional cells to carry oxygen in the blood. When the level of folic acid decreases, changes occur in the production of red cells. In the bone marrow, as the number of cells decreases, the size of the red cells increases. These large cells are different in the total hemoglobin (iron) content. These cells cannot fulfill the work of regular red cells. Red cells carry oxygen from lungs to tissues and carbon dioxide away from tissues to lungs. As a result of deficiency, several symptoms develop: tiredness, diarrhea, sore tongue, and shortness of breath, irritability, and forgetfulness. These symptoms disappear when treated with folic acid.

Requirement

The requirement for adult men and women is 2 mg. per day, but pregnant women need a little more. Lack of folic acid during pregnancy may cause mental defects in a newborn baby.

Sources

Folic acid is found in green leafy vegetables, dairy products, organ meats, and fresh fruits such as oranges and melons.

PANTOTHENIC ACID

This vitamin was discovered in 1938 and it is essential for metabolism of fat, protein, and carbohydrate. It also plays a very important role in the function of the nervous system. Lack of this vitamin causes muscular weakness, cramps, vomiting, insomnia, numbness, and prickling of the extremities. In the digestive system, lack of this vitamin may cause cancer of the colon and other digestive disorders. These symptoms quickly disappear when sufficient pantothenic acid intake is restored.

Requirement

Pantothenic acid is a water-soluble vitamin and must be supplied daily. The requirement is 7 mg. per day for adult men and women.

Sources

The major sources of this vitamin are legumes, nuts, fruits, and poultry.

VITAMIN B12

Pernicious anemia was responsible for the death of many people before the discovery of Vitamin B12. In 1948, B12 was discovered and it saved the lives of thousands of people. It is essential for the formation of DNA, protection of the sheath surrounding nerves, and the production of red blood cells. Lack of this vitamin causes a specific disease called pernicious anemia. Pernicious anemia is characterized by the release of large, immature red blood cells from the bone marrow into the blood stream. These cells are not able to carry on the work of normal red cells. The characteristics of this form of anemia are weakness, paleness, depression, confusion, and unsteadiness.

Requirement

The daily requirement for adult men and women is 3 mg. per day.

Sources

Vitamin B12 can only be found in foods of animal origin. No sources are available from plant foods. Meats such as pork, beef, poultry, seafood, and dairy products are the major sources of this vitamin.

VITAMIN C

The scientific research on Vitamin C began in 1907 when two Norwegian scientists, Holst and Frolich, produced scurvy, a deficiency disease associated with lack of Vitamin C, in guinea pigs. A British physician assigned to a ship voyaging to the "new world" conducted the first experiment on humans. During the voyage many crewmen fell ill to what we know today as scurvy. While searching for a cure, he divided his scurvy identified patients into four groups receiving vinegar, sulfuric acid, seawater, or lemon and oranges. The group receiving the lemon and oranges was cured within a short time. The other groups died. When the news arrived back in England, the British Parliament ordered that all ships leaving England on long voyages must carry limejuice and that each sailor must receive lime juice daily. For that reason, the name "limey" was given to the British sailors. Vitamin C is a water-soluble vitamin and it is not stored in the body. It requires daily intake. The excess of this vitamin is readily excreted. Vitamin C is an acid, and when combined with calcium, it produces kidney stones. Therefore, larger amounts of Vitamin C intake may contribute to the formation of kidney stones. Vitamin C is necessary for the building and maturation of bone matrix, cartilage, dentine, collagen, and connective tissue. Vascular tissue and blood vessel walls are weakened without the cementing substance of Vitamin C to provide strong capillary walls. Fragile, easily ruptured capillaries with consequent tissue bleeding characterize Vitamin C deficiency. Clinical conditions include easy bruising, easy bone fracture, poor wound healing, and bleeding gums with loosened teeth. Vitamin C plays a very important role in the production and maturation of red blood cells that is responsible for oxygen delivery to the entire tissues.

Requirement

Vitamin C can be depleted by fever and infection, stress, injury, fracture, and illness. Therefore people with stress, illness or pregnant women need to take more Vitamin C. The daily requirement is 60 mg. per day.

Sources

The best sources of Vitamin C are citrus fruits and tomatoes; however, cabbage, potatoes, green peppers, green vegetables, pineapple, broccoli, and berries can also provide a good source of this vitamin.

6

MINERALS

The invention of the electric battery in the latter part of the eighteenth century led Sir Humphrey Davey to the discovery of a number of minerals that are very important in nutrition. About 4 to 5 percent of our body weight is made up of minerals. The minerals of the body are classified into two groups.

- Minerals required in relatively larger amounts in the body are called macro-minerals.

They are:

Calcium	Sulfur
Potassium	Phosphorous
Sodium	Magnesium

- Minerals required in very small amounts are called trace minerals.

These include:
Iron
Zinc
Fluoride

Functions of Minerals

- Regulates fluid balance in the body

- Maintains acid-base balance

- Maintains nerve activities

- Maintains muscular activities

• Helps to promote growth

SALT and WEIGHT GAIN

Salt is essential for cellular function and needed only in small amounts by the body. Yet, Americans consume far more salt in their diets than do other nations. Typically excessive salt is consumed by eating processes foods, fast foods, and by adding salt during cooking or to our plates. High salt intake causes a variety of health and weight problems.

High blood pressure—excessive salt intake retains water in the body, putting pressure on blood vessels, leading to the development of high blood pressure

Joint pain—excessive salt intake causes water to accumulate in the muscles and joints

Anxiety and Depression—too much salt intake is linked to disturbance of the nervous system

Salt intake can be reduced by removing the saltshaker from the table and by substituting other spices for flavoring.

CALCIUM

The word calcium is derived from the Latin word "calx" which means chalk. Osborn and Mendel, two nutritionists, working in a laboratory, discovered that rats did not grow when they lacked calcium in their diets. They found out that the body needed calcium throughout life, especially during periods of growth, pregnancy, and lactation.

Function

• Calcium is necessary for the formation of bones and teeth

• It plays an important role in blood clotting

• It controls rhythmic beating of the heart

• It facilitates contraction of muscles

• It plays a major role in releasing energy for muscular activities

- It is needed for nerve transmission and the release of neurotransmitters at the synaptic junctions

Factors That Increase Calcium Absorption

- Vitamin D stimulates intestinal absorption of calcium

- The hydrochloric acid secreted by the stomach improves calcium absorption

- Lactose, the sugar in milk, enhances calcium absorption

- Protein. Foods high in protein accelerate calcium absorption

Factors That Reduce the Absorption of Calcium

- A diet high in fat lowers the absorption of calcium

- Vitamin D deficiency reduces calcium absorption

- Oxalic acid that is found in certain vegetables such as spinach, Swiss chard, and beets reduces the absorption of calcium

- Emotional stress influences the efficiency of calcium absorption

- Lack of exercise and especially lack of weight bearing exercises such as walking, jogging and weight lifting causes a reduction in calcium absorption

- Long term use of drugs, such as diuretics, result in decrease calcium absorption

Sources-Milk and milk products are the richest sources of calcium. If milk or milk products are not included in the daily diet, it is impossible to obtain an adequate amount of calcium. People who are lactose intolerant should use yogurt or cheese because during production lactose has been converted onto lactic acid. In other words, cheese and yogurt do not contain lactose.

Requirements-The calcium requirement is much higher during infancy than any other period of life. This higher requirement is due to the rapid rate of growth during this age. The need for calcium also increases during pregnancy and lactation. Since calcium is associated with growth, many adults feel that they do not need it, but this is not true. Calcium is very important for the normal function of the body and replacement of daily bone loss. The recommendation to meet the daily requirement is 1200 mg. per day.

OSTEOPOROSIS

This is a bone disease that occurs especially among people over 50 years of age. It is a metabolic disorder, which may be defined as a reduction in the amount of bone mass. With bone loss, the skeleton loses strength and cannot readily stand physical stress. With a minimum of physical stress, a fracture may occur. The rate of this disorder is very high among women after menopause. Osteoporosis can be detected by measuring the thickness of long bone, especially the femur, by x-ray examination.

Causes Of Osteoporosis

Osteoporosis is the result of a variety of factors:

- Lack of calcium intake during periods of growth

- Lack of absorption of calcium from the digestive system due to the aging process

- Vitamin D deficiency decreases calcium absorption

- Lack of exercise—Exercise plays a very important role in calcium metabolism, especially weight bearing exercises, such as walking, jogging, and weight training. Other exercises may develop cardiovascular fitness, but will not help in bone development.

Osteoporosis does not occur suddenly in old age, but it develops over a long period of time. Individuals complete their bone development some time within their twenties. The amount of bone attained at this point is nutritionally and genetically determined. Research suggests that the rate of bone loss after the fourth decade of life is the same among all people. That would imply that a person having less bone mass at maturity is at a higher risk for the development of osteoporosis.

Estrogen

Estrogen regulates bone mass. After menopause, the level of estrogen declines in women. This reduction in estrogen reduces the rate of calcium metabolism and weakens the bones. It is very important to notice that taking large amounts of calcium after age 50 will not prevent osteoporosis. The bones of the body must be strengthened during early age when the body is growing, by regular exercise, calcium and Vitamin D intake, so that by the time a person reaches age 50, they will have a strong bone structure. Any calcium supplement must be accompanied by Vitamin D and exercise.

IODINE

A small amount of iodine is found in the human body. Iodine is part of the thyroid hormones. It regulates body temperature, metabolic rate, and growth. The content of iodine found in food depends on the amount of iodine present in the soil where plants are grown or on which animals graze. Large amounts of iodine are found in the ocean, making seafood a good source of iodine. Since iodine is not uniformly distributed in the United States, the use of iodine salt is advisable. When the blood level of iodine is low, the cells of the thyroid gland enlarge. This is due to the synthesis of a thyroid precursor, intended to trap as many particles of iodine as possible. If the gland enlarges until it is visible, the condition is called a goiter.

Symptoms of Iodine Deficiency

- A low level of iodine produces fatigue, depression, and anxiety

- Metabolic rate goes down, as the level of iodine in the blood is lowered. As a result of low metabolic rate, body weight goes up.

- A low level of iodine also increases the level of blood cholesterol

Sources-Iodine is found in food as well as in trace amounts in drinking water. Seafood such as clams, lobsters, oysters, sardines, and other fish are major sources of iodine. Salt-water fish contains 300 to 3000 micrograms of iodine. Fresh water fish has 20 to 40 micrograms of iodine. The iodine available in the diet of the animals determines the iodine content of milk and eggs. Iodine found in vegetables is contingent upon the amount of iodine found in the soil in which they were grown.

Requirement-The National Research Council has suggested 15 mcg. per day. Pregnant or lactating women require about 25 to 50 mcg. respectively.

Deficiency

- Endemic to goiter

- Enlargement of the thyroid gland

- Low basal metabolism

- Muscular weakness

- Dry skin

- High blood cholesterol

MAGNESIUM

The importance of magnesium to the human body has only recently been emphasized. Magnesium is found in bone and in soft tissue. The body contains about 20 to 28 grams of magnesium.

Function-Magnesium is essential for the production and transfer of energy for protein synthesis, contraction of muscle, and excitability in nerves. Magnesium and calcium may have an antagonistic relationship with each other. Magnesium acts as having a relaxation role and calcium as a stimulator, therefore intake of these two minerals must be in balance. Magnesium deficiency is manifested by anorexia, growth failure, and/or neuromuscular changes. It may also produce depression and muscular weakness, tremors, and poor coordination. A deficiency in magnesium may develop by dietary inadequacy, use of diuretics, stress, and alcoholism.

Requirement-Recommendation by the National Research Council is 350 mg. per day for adult males and females. For pregnant and lactating women it is 450 mg. per day.

Sources-Magnesium is abundant in nuts, legumes, cereal, and dark green vegetables. Other sources are seafood and cocoa.

POTASSIUM

Potassium is one of the important electrolytes. Electrolytes are made up from potassium and sodium. These two minerals are responsible for initiation of nerve impulses. Disturbance of the balance between potassium and sodium produces problems such as stress, anxiety, and lack of mental awareness/alertness to the environment. This affects your ability to think clearly. Potassium contributes, along with sodium, to a normal blood pH level. It facilitates enzyme reactions related to the metabolism of protein, carbohydrate, and formation of glycogen. The level of body potassium is related to the lean body weight (muscle mass). The sudden death that occurs during severe diarrhea or fasting is thought to be due to heart failure caused by potassium deficiency. Dehydration leads to potassium loss from inside the cells. It is especially dangerous because potassium loss from brain cells makes the victim unaware of the need for water. Because of this it is advisable not to take diuretics (water pills) as the water pills cause a significant potassium loss. Diuretics should be taken only under the supervision of a physician. People working in a hot environment lose potassium through sweating they must eat more potassium-rich foods such as bananas and watermelon. Potassium tablets should not be used except under the direction of a physician. A potassium deficiency may be manifested in such conditions as vomiting, diarrhea, muscle weakness, anorexia, and edema (water retention). Other symptoms include general lack of energy, a higher pulse rate, abdominal bloating, heart rhythm abnormality, poor intestinal tone and constipation.

Requirement-Daily requirement is 50 to 150 mg. per day. People working in hot environments or athletes require more potassium.

Sources-Major sources of potassium are fruits, especially pears, prunes, bananas, and oranges. Legume sources include lima beans, pinto beans and kidney beans. Vegetable sources include potatoes, spinach, cabbage, cauliflower, broccoli and winter squash, which are rich in potassium.

FLUORIDE

The body of an average man contains 26 grams of fluoride. The average daily intake by adults is 44 mg. The fluoride content of food varies according to the content of the soil in which it was grown. Fluoride deficiency may occur at fluoride concentrations of 2 to 7 ppm. and osteoporosis at 8 to 20 ppm. In some parts of the United States, such as in the Western United States, the water sometimes contains 10 to 45 ppm. of fluoride, causing children's teeth to develop with mottled enamel. The teeth of these children are extremely resistant to tooth decay. In other areas, such as in Michigan and New York, where fluoride is deficient in the water, the incidence of dental decay is very high .One mg. of fluoride per liter of water produces a 60 to 70 percent reduction in tooth decay. Fluoride must be introduced to children at the early stages of life when teeth are forming.

In many countries where the natural fluoride content is low, fluoride is added to the drinking water.

ZINC

Zinc is known to be essential for more than 70 different enzymes. There are 1.4 to 2.3 grams of zinc in the body of an adult. The liver, pancreas, kidneys, and bones have the largest concentration of zinc.

Functions

To protect the taste buds and skin, development of sexual organs in men, and to prevent hair loss. Zinc deficiency is associated with many physiological functions, including:

- Reproductive system and growth

- Digestive system. A deficiency causes diarrhea

- It affects the immune system by making infection likely, including infection of the digestive tract

- Deficiency interferes with absorption and metabolism of Vitamin A and Folic Acid

- Other problems associated with zinc deficiency are: night blindness, thyroid disturbance, wound healing, dry skin, and alteration in taste and smell

Requirements-Recommended allowance for adults is 12 mg per day, but the RDA recommends 18 mg per day for adults and 5 to 6 mg additional during pregnancy. Excessive intake of zinc causes diarrhea, vomiting, anemia, dizziness, and kidney failure.

Sources-Animal products and legumes are good sources of zinc, such as liver, eggs, and lean meat.

SODIUM

People throughout history appreciated the nutritional value of sodium. Some practical uses of sodium, commonly known as salt, include seasoning, a food preservative, and wound cleanser. Additionally, it is a very important nutrient and necessary for all functions of the body. The distribution of water in the body depends on the location and concentration of sodium and potassium. Muscles and nerve activities are all regulated by sodium and potassium. The activities of the kidneys regulate the blood sodium level. If the level of blood sodium drops below the normal range it causes anxiety, fatigue and fast pulse rate. The level of blood sodium drops during vomiting, diarrhea and heavy sweating. On the other hand, if the blood sodium level goes up it causes water retention, high blood pressure, and lack of energy. During heavy sweating, vomiting and extensive sunburn, both water and sodium must be replenished to prevent medical problems from occurring. If only water is provided, the blood concentration of sodium will drop and symptoms of water intoxication can occur such as headache, poor memory, and weakness. Sodium constitutes two percent of the total minerals in the body. It is involved in three major physiological functions:

- Maintenance of normal water balance

- Maintenance of acid-base balance in the body

- Maintenance of normal nerve and muscular transmission activities

If the blood concentration of sodium rises, as it will after a person eats a salty meal, the thirst mechanism ensures that a person will desire to drink water until the water balance is adjusted. A high intake of sodium causes water retention in the body. The water retention not only causes fatigue, irritation and sleep disturbance, but it also raises blood pressure. High salt intake is very dangerous to pregnant women. It increases blood pressure and also causes problems for the newborn. Therefore, pregnant women should be told to restrict their salt intake throughout pregnancy. Low blood sodium has its own serious problems as well. When the level of blood sodium drops, as during vomiting, heavy sweating, and diarrhea, it causes muscular cramps, fatigue, rapid pulse, and low blood pressure.

Requirements-In the United States, the consumption of salt is very high. It is about10 to 18 grams per day. The average recommended sodium intake is 4 to 6 grams per day. One reason for higher consumption of salt is that Americans use more processed foods such as prepackaged foods and foods sold in jars and cans, which are very high in salt concentration.

CHROMIUM

The concentration of chromium is higher during infancy than other periods of life. Concentrations of chromium in the tissues decrease steadily with increasing age.

Functions-Chromium plays a very important role in glucose metabolism. Chromium deficiency is characterized by inability to metabolize glucose, slow growth, and lack of energy, fatigue, and peripheral neuropathy. Chromium reduces the cholesterol ratio, which is a protective index for the rate of cardiovascular diseases.

Deficiency of Chromium

- Reduces the production of insulin

- Lowers the production of energy from glucose

- Causes diabetes

Sources—major sources of chromium are potatoes, vegetable oils, and whole-wheat products.

Requirement—the requirement of chromium is 50 to 200 mcgs for normal adults.

PHOSPHORUS

Phosphorus makes up one percent of the body weight and 85 percent of it is found with calcium in the bones and teeth. It is the chief compound that gives teeth and bone strength and rigidity. Phosphorus is also part of DNA, the genetic code material present in every cell in the body. It is necessary for growth and development of the tissues. Phosphorus is one of the essential minerals. It comprises 22 percent of the total minerals in the body. Most phosphorus is located in the bones and teeth and the rest of this mineral is found in the extra-cellular fluid.

Functions—this mineral has several important functions in the body:

- It is a key component in the structure of cell membranes

- It plays an important role in the metabolic process involving protein, carbohydrate, and fat, and also in the production of energy

- Phosphorus with calcium is necessary for nerve transmission and muscular contraction

Sources—animal foods such as meat, fish, poultry, milk, and eggs are the best sources of this mineral. Phosphorus is also found in grains and cereal.

Requirements—the daily requirement of phosphorus is almost the same as that of calcium for all age groups. It is 800 to 900 mg per day.

IRON

The role of iron in the blood seems to hold peculiar fascination for Americans. Television and newspapers are telling women that they must take iron everyday and that they need more iron than men. Historically, iron was discovered in the nineteenth century. It was thought that iron was part of human blood. Most of the iron in the body is a component of the proteins hemoglobin and myoglobin. Both these components carry oxygen in association with iron. They contain hemoglobin as the oxygen carrier in red cells and myoglobin as the receiver in the muscle cells. All cells use oxygen and nutrients to keep pathways open for the constant release of energy. The red cells shuttle between metabolizing tissues and lungs to bring in fresh oxygen supplies. Iron deficiency has been cited as the most common of all deficiency diseases in both developing and under developed countries. The groups considered the most frequently at risk are children under two years of age, teenagers, pregnant women, and the elderly. Iron deficiency manifests itself by the development of anemia. It can be corrected by consuming a diet rich in iron and by providing iron supplements in the form of ferrous sulfate or ferrous glutamate. Sulfate ferrous glutamate iron deficiency can be caused by loss of blood and degenerative diseases that interfere with iron absorption.

Functions—Iron plays a very important role in the production of red blood cells. When the level of iron goes down, the red cells will contain too little hemoglobin. They become unable to carry enough oxygen to meet the cells needs. Iron deficiency symptoms are:

- Lack of energy, lack of sleep, emotional stress

- Low learning ability, lack of competence, short memory, and poor attention span

- Dry and itchy skin

- Infection. Iron deficiency has been shown to reduce the body's resistance

- Lack of iron causes general fatigue, anemia and pain in the bones

Requirement—the daily allowance for iron is 18 mg per day. For women it is a little more. It is important that iron should be obtained from food sources rather than through supplementation. Iron from fortified foods and from supplements is poorly absorbed even though they may contain as much as 50 mg of iron per day. Cooking utensils can enhance the amount of iron. The iron content of 100 grams of meat simmered in a glass dish is 3 mg, however when it is cooked in an iron skillet it becomes 8 mg. You can triple the iron content of a scrambled egg by cooking it in an iron pan. Foods containing 25 mg of Vitamin C can double the amount of iron absorbed.

Factors that enhance iron absorption

Vitamin C—the effect of Vitamin C on iron absorption is widely accepted. It is now recommended that iron be accompanied by the intake of Vitamin C.

Animal protein—not all protein enhances the absorption of iron, only a cellular protein such as beef, pork, veal, lamb, liver, fish, and cow's milk can enhance iron absorption.

Human milk—infants retain more iron from human milk than from cow's milk or infant formula.

Calcium—the presence of an adequate amount of calcium in the diet helps to increase iron absorption.

Factors that Decrease Iron Absorption

- Lack of hydrochloric acid in the stomach

- Administration of alkaline substances such as antacids interferes with iron absorption.

Source-The richest sources of iron are liver and pork, with liver containing the highest amount and chicken liver containing the lowest amount. Other meat products such as organ meats and eggs are good sources of iron.

Green leafy vegetables and dried fruits make a good contribution. The rule of thumb is, the greener the vegetable, the higher the iron content.

MINERAL TOXICITY

Minerals can be extremely toxic and cause serious problems. Special attention must be given to the trace minerals. Mineral supplements exceeding 1.5 times the recommendation should be taken only under medical supervision. Trace minerals most likely to cause toxicity are.

Iron—a large dosage of iron supplement can be life threatening. Iron pills and vitamin supplements that contain iron can poison children. Excessive iron deposited in tissues causes severe liver and heart damage.

Zinc—high dosage of zinc interferes with iron and copper absorption. A zinc supplement taken at three times its requirement reduces good cholesterol in the blood by 15 percent. By taking a zinc supplement you may be increasing you risk for developing heart disease.

Selenium—over intake of selenium is associated with hair loss, weakness, rashes and cirrhosis of the liver.

Iodine—high intake of iodine disturbs the function of the thyroid gland. This can occur in people who eat a lot of seaweed. Seaweed is very high in iodine.

Fluoride—high fluoride intake can mottle teeth during their development. It also weakens the tooth structure.

7

WATER

Water in the human body is like a river crossing through the arteries, capillaries and veins carrying a heavy load of nutrients and waste products. Water is in every part of the body including the cells, bones, tissues, skin, and ligaments. From 55 to 65 percent of the body is made up of water. Water molecules are also found inside proteins, glycogen, and in other macromolecules of the body, helping to form their structure. A little alteration in the water content of the body can cause dehydration, shock, and death.

Function—water serves many functions.

- Water serves as a building material for growth and repair in the body

- Water plays an important role in digestion, absorption, and excretion

- It acts as a transport medium for nutrients and all body substances

- Water carries the metabolic waste produced in the cells and excretes it through the urine

- Fiber and cellulose in food absorb water and aids in the elimination of fecal residue

- Water maintains body temperature

- Water acts as lubrication in the joints. Without water, joints cannot function properly.

- Water serves as a shock absorber inside the eyes, spinal cord, heart, kidneys, and liver. It protects the vital organs of the body. The body can survive a deficiency of all other nutrients for a long time, but it can survive only a few days without water, because the body must excrete a minimum amount of water each day, carrying the waste products generated by metabolic process.

Water Balance—the water content of the fat free body weight remains fairly constant by homoeostatic regulations. This is a result of the interaction among antidiuretic hormones, the gastrointestinal tract, the kidneys, and the brain. The amount of water taken in daily is equal to the amount of water loss.

Water Intake—water intake is controlled by thirst sensation. The thirst control centers are located in the hypothalamus. Thirst is stimulated when the water volume of the body decreases or receptors in the great vessels are affected.

Sources of Water—most adults consume 1.5 to 2 liters of water daily through drinks and foods, plus water from the oxidation of food in the body.

- Daily fluid intake provides 500 to 1500 ml of water

- Daily food intake provides 800 to 1000 ml of water

- Cellular oxidation of foods provides 200 to 300 ml of water daily

Thirst and satiety govern water intake. When the blood is too concentrated it solutes attract water out of the salivary glands and the mouth becomes dry. As a result, you drink to wet your mouth. The brain center becomes involved because the hypothalamus also monitors the salt concentration of the blood. When the salt concentration of the blood is too high, the hypothalamus initiates impulses that stimulate drinking behavior.

Water elimination—there are four ways in which the body eliminates water.

- Water is lost from the lungs as we expire air

- Water is lost from the kidneys as urine. Normally an adult excretes 600 to 1600 ml of urine per day.

- Water is lost through perspiration

- Water is lost through the bowel in the feces

Abnormal water loss occurs through vomiting, diarrhea, and hemorrhages. The body has no place to store water. Water must be replaced on a daily basis in order to maintain a healthy water balance.

Water Requirement—according to the Food and Nutrition Board, a daily water intake of 2.5 liters or 3 quarts of water is needed to carry on the essential activities of the body. Special attention should be given to adults or infants who are on protein diets, to people in hot environments, or to those who have high fever and/or diarrhea.

8

CHOLESTEROL

How to lower cholesterol

Cholesterol is a fatty substance found in the blood and in the membrane of nervous tissues. Cholesterol is very important for the proper functioning of the nervous system. It also protects the body against radiation.

Cholesterol comes from two sources—foods we consume and from the liver. The liver produces cholesterol mostly from carbohydrate foods.

What is a normal cholesterol level?

Cholesterol has two components

- High-density cholesterol

- Low-density cholesterol

The overall cholesterol level should range from 150-200 mg/100cc
High-density cholesterol should range from 50-70 mg/100cc
Low-density cholesterol should be less than 130 mg/100cc

Cholesterol levels that are more than 200 may hasten a very serious problem in the occurrence of cardiovascular disease. Excessive cholesterol deposits in the walls of the arteries reduces blood flow to the heart and other organs in the body.

High Cholesterol Foods

Cholesterol is found in animal products. Plants do not have any cholesterol.
Animal Sources include meats, eggs, dairy products (butter, milk, cheese, cottage cheese), shellfish, and fried foods.

Foods Without Cholesterol

They include fish (any variety), chicken cutlet, turkey breast, fruits, vegetables, legumes, potato, bread, pasta, and cereal. Regarding pasta, it does not contain cholesterol per se, but will be converted by your body to cholesterol if consumed too frequently.

Sample of a low-cholesterol weekly diet

Breakfast—select one

Fruit, Cereal with skim milk, toast with jam, low fat yogurt with a fruit, bagel with jam, oatmeal.

Lunch—select one

Salad with turkey, salad with an apple, grilled chicken with salad, tuna fish sandwich, yogurt with a fruit.

Dinner—select one

Tooshi's Dinner w/chicken, steamed chicken with steamed vegetables, steamed fish with steamed vegetables, grilled chicken with salad.
Note: If you do not need to lose weight you can have potato or rice with your dinners, but not pasta until your cholesterol levels have improved.

Low-cholesterol dinner options

Tooshi's Dinner	Mediterranean Delight
French Delight	Chicken Cutlet
Stuffed Flounder	Stuffed Pepper (substitute turkey)
Fish La Chanta	Food for Heart

Meatball Dinner (substitute turkey)
Steamed fish with steamed vegetables
Steamed chicken with steamed vegetables

Physical Exercise

Physical exercise plays a very important role in reducing blood cholesterol but exercise must have a special intensity and duration to affect the metabolism of cholesterol. Only certain types of exercise can reduce cholesterol.

They are: walking, jogging, cross country skiing, cycling, and swimming.

Intensity—is based on pulse rate to be effective. Exercise pulse rates should be between 130-140 beats per minute.

Duration—of exercise must be between 45-60 minutes per day.

Frequency—should be at least 5-6 times per week.

9

BODY COMPOSITION AND BODY TYPE

Observation shows that people come in different shapes, heights and weights. Some are slim, or tall, or short, or fat and overweight. The question arises: what are the causes of these different body types? Are they basically genetic or environmental? Genetically, each person has 46 chromosomes. Twenty-three of them come from the father and the other 23 come from the mother. These chromosomes contain DNA, which is the building block of the genetic characteristics of people. These DNA carry characteristics of the mother and the father to the newborn baby, which includes shape, height and psychological makeup of both parents. It is true that children are the product of both genetic and environmental factors. However, the environment cannot change the shape and body type from what was inherited but how you live in the environment might.

When a female egg and male sperm combine, they produce a fertilized egg. This egg contains 46 chromosomes with half belonging to the mother. The other half belongs to the father. The fertilized egg begins to grow and becomes a mass of cells, which is the start of an embryo. The embryo grows and divides into three sections. These sections are: The Outer Layer, The Middle Layer, and The Inner Layer. The outer layer cells grow and produce the skin, nose, ears, and sexual organs of the male, fingers, and toes. The middle layer cells grow and produce muscles and the skeletal system. The inner layer grows and produces the stomach, intestines and organs.

During the embryonic stage, if any one of these three layers dominates the growth, the individual will have characteristics of either ectomorpic, mesomorphic, or endomorphic. For example, if the outer layer dominates the other two, the person becomes ectomorphic, that means slim and trim looking but not muscular. If the middle section dominates growth, the person will have very strong muscles and bones. If the inner section grows more than the other two, the per-

81

son becomes overweight, with a large amount of adipose tissue and a larger digestive system.

Personality of body types

Ectomorphs, genetically, have a very low appetite, not very strong body structure, are psychologically fearful, do not have very much confidence, and tend to have a less efficient immune system. They have a very high tendency for having emotional stress. Usually they hide their feelings and do not reveal their thoughts to the outside world. This group is sometimes called personality Type C and is prone to suicide. Most suicide victims come from this group.

Mesomorphics are physically very strong, emotionally ambitious, are confident, have a high self-image, and are strong leaders with dominant characteristics, who live to dominate others. Yet genetically they are born with poor cardiovascular systems. They die from heart disease early if they become inactive and sedentary. For them to extend their longevity, they must:

- Participate in regular cardiovascular activity

- Monitor their body weight

- Reduce saturated fat in their diets

Extensive weight lifting may play a negative role in promoting cardiovascular health. This Group is called Type A Personality.

Endomorphics are the people born with the tendency to gain weight because of having a large digestive system. They eat more, have large appetites and consume large portions. Psychologically they are calm, sociable, but have little confidence in themselves, little ambition and live shorter lives. These people are genetically unable to lose weight because of the large digestive system derived from the embryonic stage. They consume more food than the other two groups. Since physiological growth ends at the age of 18 to 22, nothing substantial can be done to help them to lose weight but any weight gain after age 22 can be reduced by proper diet and regular physical activity. This group is called Personality Type B.

If an overweight person marries another overweight person, the chances that their children will be overweight are 80%. But if an overweight person marries an average weight person, the chance the offspring will be overweight is now 40%. The question is, where is the missing 20%? Studies show the gene of the grandparents may skip a generation and if they are overweight, the newborn has a 20% chance to become overweight. However if they are average weight, the newborn has a 20% chance to become average weight.

Sheldon, a psychologist, came out with a perspective and a triangular diagram placing the three body type extremes on each angle. He believed that through genetics, the three body types might slide towards each other. For example, endomorphic becomes Endo-Meso or mesomorphic becomes Meso-Endo and ectomorphic becomes Ecto-Meso. He hypothesized that regular physical exercise and proper nutrition can play a role in influencing body type appearance. Ectomorphics can gain 20-25 percent of the characteristics of mesomorphics and lose 20 to 25 percent of the ectomorphic characteristic. Mesomorphics through sedentary living and poor nutrition will gain 20-25 percent of mesomorphic character and gain 20-25 percent of the endomorohic character. Endomorphics can gain 20-25 percent of mesomorphic character and 20-25 percent of mesomorphic character if they participate in only regular cardiovascular exercise, eat a proper diet and reduce the portion of the food they consume.

How to measure your body weight

Various formal and informal scales tell you what your ideal weight should be. Some of these scales are very confusing, as not everyone's frames are the same. People come in all shapes, some small, some medium, and others are larger. To calculate your ideal weight you should follow the scale below.

Ideal weight for women

If a woman is 4 feet 10 inches tall and has one of the following frames, her ideal weight would be:

Frame	Weight
Small	95 lbs
Medium	105 lbs
Large	115 lbs

If a woman is taller than 4 feet 10 inches, add 3 pounds for every inch above 4 feet, 10 inches. For example, the ideal weight for a medium frame woman at 5 feet, 5 inches tall will be according to the following formula:

5 feet 5 inches minus 4 feet 1 inch equals 7 inches	(5'5' - 4'1" = 7)
7 times 3 equals 21	(7 x 3 = 21)
21 plus 105 equals 126	(21 + 105 = 126)

Therefore, a woman 5 feet 5 inches tall with a medium frame should weigh 126 pounds.

Ideal weight for men

Men also come with small, medium, or larger frames. The ideal weight for a man 5 feet 2 inches in height would be:

Frame	Weight
Small	115 lbs
Medium	136 lbs
Large	145 lbs

Add 4 pounds for every inch above 5'2". For example, the ideal weight for a man with a larger frame would be according to the following formula:

5 feet 10 inches minus 5 feet 2 inches equals 8 inches	(5'10" - 5'2" = 8)
8 times 4 equals 32	(8 x 4=32)
145 plus 32 equals 177	(145 + 32 = 177)

Therefore, a man 5 feet 10 inches tall with a large frame should weigh 177 pounds.

Proper eating habits

Physical exercise without proper eating habits cannot contribute very much to your total health. The ability to select good foods plays a very important role in good performance of the athlete events. A balanced diet should be comprised from carbohydrates, proteins, and fats.

Carbohydrates: As mentioned in a previous chapter, carbohydrates come from plant foods. Some of those foods promote health and energize the body, whereas others have very little effect on health and well being. Good carbohydrates are divided into starches and fruit.

Starches. Starches can include rice, potatoes, whole grain, and rye.

Fruits. It is good to select and consume seasonal fruits.
In spring, select strawberries and blueberries.
In summer, consume apples, grapes, peaches, watermelon, and cantaloupe.
During winter, choose orange, grapefruit, banana, and pineapple.
Avoid frozen, canned, and jarred fruits. These sources contain added sugar, salt, chemicals, and other preservatives. Carbohydrates that should be avoided are: Cookies, pies, candy, white bread, white pasta, muffins and cakes.

Proteins. There are three kinds of proteins:

Animal protein such as beef, pork, chicken, turkey, and seafood

Animal by-products. Eggs and Dairy Products such as milk, cheese, yogurt, butter and ice cream

Plant protein, such as legumes and complex carbohydrates
Athletes should consume more seafood including fish, shrimp, and scallops but less beef or pork. Eggs, low fat milk, cheese and yogurt will provide great amounts of good protein and calcium. Legumes and complex carbohydrates are good sources of plant protein and should be included in your daily diet.

Fats. Fats contain very high calories. Effort should be made to use plant fats such as corn oil and olive oil. Fats derived from animal products such as butter and mayonnaise cause high blood cholesterol and heart disease. Margarine, which looks like butter is converted from plant oils. According to research studies, margarine may cause cancer because of the high temperature used in the production of margarine-based products.

Liquids. Water plays an important role in the body. Without water no chemical activities take place in the body. The best liquid to satisfy thirst is water. Other drinks such as soft drinks contain salt and other chemicals, which will have a negative effect on energy. Coffee or tea must be used in moderation, since coffee and tea contain caffeine. Caffeine may lower blood sugar and cause fatigue. Consumption of more than three cups per day will have a negative effect on athletic performance.

Daily athletic diet

Breakfast is an essential part of the diet. No one should miss breakfast. Breakfast provides energy to the body and keeps the blood sugar in normal range without fluctuation.
Breakfast should consist of the following options:
Two soft-boiled eggs with two slices of rye bread and a glass of milk
Low salt, low sugar cereal with 1% milk and a banana or raisins
Two slices of rye bread and two slices of alpine lace cheese with a glass of milk

Lunch:

Turkey sandwich (two slices rye bread, ¼ pound low salt turkey breast, lettuce and tomato)
Salad with grilled chicken
Tuna fish sandwich (rye bread, lettuce, tomato, but no mayonnaise)

Dinner:

Fish with a variety of fresh vegetables, rice, and salad
Chicken cutlet with fresh vegetables, potato and salad
Seafood with pasta, vegetables and salad
Steak, lean beef or pork should not be used more than once a week
You may substitute frozen vegetables but not canned vegetables.

Snacks:

The best snacks are fruit. Athletes should eat at least 3 to 4 fresh fruits per day. A variety of fruits should be eaten rather than the same fruits. Effort should be made to avoid too much salt and fats. It is good practice not to order from the menu when you eat out. You always have the option to order what you want. The food options on the menu are very high in fat and salt. It is better to tell the waiter how you want your meal prepared. More often than not, restaurants have all the ingredients available and the means to be flexible.

Alcohol:

Consumption of alcohol should be occasionally rather than every day.

Dinner Time:

The time of eating dinner is very important. If dinner is eaten early such as 5 or 6 PM you will be left with lots of time before going to bed. The chances that you are going to snack after dinner are very high. The best hours to eat dinner are between 7 and 9 PM.

Desserts:

Pie, ice cream, cake, muffins and sugary snack foods should only be eaten occasionally.

Dried Foods:

Dried foods such as raisins, dates, figs etc. are excellent sources of carbohydrates, minerals, and vitamins.

Nuts:

Nuts provide a good amount of proteins, carbohydrates and good fats. They are good sources of vitamins and minerals.

Athletes should include nuts such as walnuts and almonds in their diets. These nuts may prevent cancer.

TOOSHI'S LAW: *"A Slim Chance and A Fat Chance Mean the Same.*

PART III
THE PHYSIOLOGICAL BENEFITS OF EXERCISE

10

THE PHYSIOLOGICAL BENEFITS OF EXERCISE

This chapter provides you with a basic understanding of human physiology and outlines the physical effects exercise has on the body, the benefits gained through physical training, and the benefits exercise produces in your body.

The Human Machine

Our body is a magnificent machine designed for movement like other machines. It has an engine, which uses fuel and produces energy needed for daily activities, including the activities of our heart, lungs, kidneys, brain and activities of other organs. Our engine has a pump—the heart—that circulates blood, a wiring network—the vascular system—to deliver blood nutrients and heat to every corner of the body. It has a ventilation system—the lungs—that takes fresh air into the body and removes toxic air to the outside. Our fuel conversion center—called metabolism—converts our food energy into mechanical and electrical energy needed for physical activity and neurological activities.

Let us take a journey inside this machine and see how various parts of it work. First let us stop at the pumping station (the heart), to check its beating frequency (pulse rate) to see if it beats fast or slow or just right. Then on to check the pressure produced during each beat (blood pressure) to see if it is normal, high or low. We also need to check the volume of blood ejected during each heartbeat. If the heart is ejecting more blood you should feel energetic or "up" but if the ejection volume is low you tend to feel tired or "down."

Our second stop will be the wiring network—vascular system—to see if our wires are clean, without deposits or buildups inside and that the blood circulates smoothly.

The third stop is the ventilation center—the lungs—to check if our breathing is deep, shallow or just right at 16 respirations per minute. Then we observe the fuel conversion processes. The types of fuel used—the foods we eat. The efficiency of the energy produced: are we feeling tired, weak (bad fuels/poor diet) or feeling good, energetic and happy (good fuel/good diet).

Finally, we end our journey at the waste-producing center—the kidneys and digestive system. We check the color and volume of urine and feces produced. We check to see if we have any malfunctions regarding bowel discomfort, stomach pain, bloatedness, gas, or constipation. The kidneys and digestive system remove the metabolic waste of food. The quality of our lives is based on the performance of this remarkable machine. We must do everything in our power to keep it in top working order by:

- Providing the best clean and high efficiency fuels (food)

- Maintaining and improving system efficiency through regular physical exercise

- Avoiding toxic material buildup through quick and efficient removal of metabolic wastes, which are linked to some cancers and chronic diseases.

It is extremely important for us to learn and understand the working processes of our bodies because we don't come into this world with an owner's manual so to speak. Any problems we notice in our bodies are warning signs, such as weakness, fatigue, pain, sleeping problems, emotional stress, constipation, stomach pain, acid reflux, or bad mood. All of these problems are related in one way to poor eating habits and poor metabolic processes. From this journey we should learn three important lessons. First, to keep every part of our bodies in good working condition and lasting for a longer time by providing clean and efficient fuel (proper diet). Secondly, we must keep ourselves physically active throughout life (regular exercise). And thirdly, providing clean air by avoiding toxic environments and smoking.

TOOSHI'S LAW: *"You don't control the roads, just your own vehicle."*

The effects of exercise on the mind and body

If you sit too much and spend hours on your feet, you may find yourself at risk for blood clotting, especially in your leg extremities. Sometimes clots break off and travel to the lungs, heart, or brain causing death. Anyone who does not get enough physical exercise to maintain adequate circulation in the legs can become susceptible to blood clots as they age. Typically professions such as teachers, policemen, firemen, bus and cab drivers, and anyone bedridden are prone to vascular disease. There are some things you can do to prevent vascular disease–stretch every hour, lose weight, or take short walks. Physical exercise increases a protein substance in the body that helps dissolve blood clots and reduces the chances of clot formation. Excessive salt intake contributes to water retention and causes tightening and narrowing of arteries. Tightening and narrowing of the arteries increases blood pressure and may lead to rupture of the small blood vessels within the brain. Aerobic exercise increases a chemical called TPA in the blood that helps to lower blood pressure and increase high-density cholesterol.

There is something very satisfying about using your body the way nature intended it to be used. In this complicated, fast-paced world, filled with distraction, tension, and unrest, the gratifying release exercise offers appears, for many, to be one of the best natural sources of tranquility. Ask anyone who exercises regularly and you will see how daily exercise can transform a sedentary, arm-chair thinker or sullen and depressed individual into an energetic, active, passionate doer. Thoughts are biochemical reactions. Our mental outlook is influenced by how we feel. Today, we must get out of our easy-chairs, away from our TV sets, out of our cars, our cubicles, and our daily grind. Taking advantage of the opportunities our health centers, grasslands, parks, and roads offer can provide exercise and reactivate our mind-body link. Exercising outside has a restorative effect on the nervous system by refreshing your mind and spirit, helping to relieve stress, and bring back lost energy. A true sense of well-being surely depends upon the right use of the physiological machine, which is so much a part of who we are and how we feel. Indeed, we owe it to ourselves to care for our bodies by exercising because they were designed to move.

We are concerned primarily with:

- The Onset of Exercise (Getting Started)

- The Long-Term Effects of Exercise (Training Effect)

In order to truly study the physiological effects of exercise on the body and the benefits gained by physical training it is essential to have an understanding of the relevant changes exercise produces in the various parts of our bodies and a knowledge of basic human physiology. One must be familiar with the way the cardiovascular and respiratory systems work, with the basic mechanism of muscular contraction, and the principles behind the development of strength and endurance. Understanding your system and its present capacity is very important prior to undertaking a serious exercise program.

Structure and function of cells

All living organisms are made up from cells. Cells are regarded as the unit of living material. Studying cells, their forms and functions is called cytology. Cytologists are interested in the processes within the cells, namely the contents, needs, and functions of cells.

There are many varieties of cells depending where they are located. The bones, heart, liver, kidneys, and lungs, for example, all have different cells and they each have specific functions. Heart cells contract and push blood out of the heart. The cells of the nervous system conduct impulses. However, all cells regardless of location have an outside cover called a membrane. The membrane contains many small holes where the exchange of water and nutrients occur. Inside each cell are cytoplasm, a substance containing water, protein, and genetic material called DNA.

Each of our body's organs is made up from a group of cells. These cells are designed to serve that particular organ, but with each group performing a different function specific to the organ they serve. For example, some cells secrete enzymes and other cells send impulses. But, all cells require water, protein, carbohydrate, fat, vitamins, minerals, and oxygen and all cells release metabolic waste.

A diet low in fat and containing more fruits and vegetables plays a very important role in proper cellular functioning. A good diet not only increases the release of energy, but it also prevents premature aging of cells. To increase the oxygen intake and lung capacity we also need to engage in regular cardiovascular exercise optimally at 45 minutes a day, five days a week and minimally, at 30 minutes a day, three days a week.

11

EFFECTS OF EXERCISE ON THE CARDIOVASCULAR SYSTEM

Exercise and Weight Loss

Fat is deposited under the skin, between tissues, and inside muscle. Fat serves several functions in the body including:

Reducing the loss of body heat

Serving as a reserve fuel supply

Energy production

Acting as a cushion around major organs—such as the heart, kidney, liver, and lungs

Despite the beneficial attributes of fat, serious health risks may occur when large amounts of fat accumulate in the body. Life insurance companies have indicated that overweight people are more prone to heart disease, high blood pressure, high cholesterol, shorter life expectancy, a thirty percent higher death rate for being 15-20 pounds overweight, and an 80 percent higher death rate for being as much as 35 pounds or more overweight. Diseases related to heart attack and poor circulation are associated with obesity. High blood pressure and hardening of the arteries are three times higher among those considered obese. Overweight people have more muscle and joint ailments. Even respiratory problems are attributed to excessive weight.

Physical exercise plays a very important role in combating obesity. Exercise increases metabolism, reduces appetite, helps burn calories, improves circulation, raises body temperature, and lowers blood pressure and blood sugar. Above all, exercise helps control body weight, creates confidence, self-control, a positive self-image, and slows down the aging process. Exercising more vigorously has been linked to combating emotional stress. Regular exercise enhances the transit process of blood sugar into the cells, lowering blood sugar and reducing the need for insulin production. Exercise helps reduce the LDL cholesterol while increasing the HDL cholesterol. Tremendous benefit fighting obesity can be gained from walking, jogging, or cycling just thirty to forty minutes a day, three times per week as 400-500 calories are burned with each work session. Another aspect to keep in mind is that exercise serves to reduce your appetite.

Cardiac output and endurance training

Exercise strengthens the heart muscle, especially when one is engaged in an activity such as endurance training. The result is an increased stroke volume, made possible by the heart emptying its contents more quickly than it occurs in the untrained state. In a trained state the heart beats less frequently both at rest and during comparative workloads, but because of other circulatory changes accompanying the training, more physical work can be accomplished. The ability of a conditioned athlete's heart to pump blood and oxygen to the tissues is much greater than that of a non-athlete. Therefore an athlete can accomplish much more physical work with greater ease.

Endurance training enlarges the heart. The enlargement occurring in this case differs from an enlarged heart in sedentary people. Sedentary living atrophies the thickness of the muscle wall of the heart and reduces blood volume as well as the heart's pumping action.

The enlarged heart of an individual accustomed to endurance training possesses:

- Stronger pumping force

- Higher stroke volume

- Slower pulse rate

- Higher capacity for long-term physical work

- Increased strength of contraction

Coronary Circulation

Due to the crucial role that the heart plays in physical exercise, the heart has attracted a great deal of attention from both medical professionals and the general public. Heart disease often leads to physical inactivity because patients are typically instructed to limit their physical activity, let alone engage themselves actively in exercise. Ironically, the resulting lack of exercise brings about further deterioration of the muscles due to reduced circulation. The heart, like all other muscles, requires adequate blood flow to function normally.

Blood circulation to the heart is supplied by the right and left coronary arteries, both of which arise from the aorta. The coronary arteries infiltrate the myocardium, extending into branches and forming a complete circulatory network. Endurance training increases the flow of blood through the coronary vessels. Collateral circulation is important in preventing a heart attack. Collateral circulation is a new blood vessel, which is produced as a result of endurance training.

Considerable research has been undertaken to understand the effects of training on the cardiovascular system and, in particular, on the heart itself. Activities such as running, swimming, cycling, and cross-country skiing have been shown to lead to significant improvements in circulation and the functioning of the heart. Strength training exercises such as weight lifting, in contrast, tax the body's aerobic capacity. Weight training is not generally conducive to improving the cardiovascular system.

Aerobic exercise, known as "steady rate performance," can be continued for long periods of time since the rate of energy expenditure is equal to that of oxygen intake. When the rate of energy expenditure is greater than the oxygen intake, the steady rate is exceeded and maximum exercise occurs, resulting in a buildup of lactic acid. The buildup of lactic acid that accompanies maximum exercise is an early sign of oxygen debt development. Most people experience lactic acid build up and muscular cramp as fatigue about two days after exercising.

Heart Rate

Physical training reduces the heart's resting rate. A larger stroke volume, more efficient circulation, and a greater absorption of oxygen from the blood by the tissues accompany the slower resting rate. A conditioned athlete enjoys a slower heart rate for any given workload when compared with his or her non-trained counterpart. A lower resting pulse rate among trained people is related to:

- Decreased intrinsic firing of the S.A. node

- Increased parasympatic nerve activity, which helps to relax the body

- Larger stroke volume

TOOSHI'S LAW: *"Use It or Lose It."*

12

SHORT TERM EFFECT OF EXERCISE ON THE HEART

TOOSHI'S LAW: *"Age is Irrelevant."*

The heart is comprised of muscle tissue like other muscles but it differs in four important ways:

- The activity of the heart muscle never ceases, even under conditions of rest

- The oxygen consumption of the heart resembles that of the skeletal muscles during exercise

- The heart is distinguished by the fact that its oxygen need does not change significantly during physical activity

- The heart utilizes glucose for its metabolism as well as lactic acid and pyretic acid obtained directly from the blood

Factors affecting the heart during exercise
Age

It should be clearly realized that chronological age is not necessarily a significant factor, but physiological and psychological age can play an important role in an individual's capacity for exercise. Regarding maximal work, fitness is a much more important factor than one's chronological age.

Gender

There are marked differences between the physiological capacities of men and women regarding their ability to perform hard exercise. Differences in stroke volume play an important role in one's capacity for exercise: stroke volume measures

209 ml for men and 161 ml for women. Maximum cardiac output is another important factor: it measures 37 liters in men and 25 liters in women. For a given work load, the heart rate is higher in women than men. In addition, the oxygen content of the blood is higher in men than in women on average, allowing for men to perform more and harder exercise than their female counterparts.

Fitness

An individual's fitness constitutes the most important factor determining the level of cardiovascular reaction to exercise. Studies show that among healthy individuals of similar age, marked differences exist in the ability to perform physical work and to recover from it. An individual variability exists at the physiological level for a variety of physical work, at rest, during exercise, and at recovery for moderate work and during and after hard exercise.

A fit person is able to maintain a slower heart rate at work and recover from standard work better than a less fit individual. The basis for measuring an individual's capacity for physical work should focus upon that person's ability to perform the activity as well as their speed of recovery.

Effects of exercise on the muscular system

Physical training, if performed regularly, produces an increase in the size of the skeletal muscles. This muscular hypotrophy is not, however, related to the formation of new muscle fibers, but to the growth and development of existing fibers. When regular exercise places greater demands upon the muscles, muscle fibers develop to their full size. The increase in size is accompanied by the development of expanded capillary networks in the trained muscles. Strength exercise, such as weightlifting and isometric exercises, generally produces a hypotrophy of the fibers. Endurance exercise, however, such as running, swimming, and cycling, lead to an increase in the number of capillaries in the muscles.

In light of these factors, the following questions arise:

What is strength?

Strength refers to one's ability to produce more powerful muscular contractions, which generate the greater force needed to lift heavier loads.

What is endurance?

Endurance refers to one's ability to repeat muscular contractions over a long duration of time. Running for a long distance is a common example of an endurance-testing activity.

What is speed?

Speed refers to one's ability to repeat muscular contractions rapidly.

Exercising the muscles against progressively greater resistance can develop muscle strength. The increase in resistance must be a gradual process, however, lifting weights, pulling a spring, or pushing a stationary object are common examples of strength-developing exercises. A gain in strength means more than simply muscular hypotrophy; i.e., growth in size, as it is possible to increase strength without increasing the size of the muscles. Weight training can increase strength without increasing size of the muscles.

Muscular reactions to training vary. The kind of exercise being performed matters, as does the intensity of contraction. The degrees of repetition, speed, and duration are also important. Again, strength does not necessarily imply gains in speed and endurance. Increased vascularization in trained muscle provides more oxygen and more fuel for the muscular system so that muscles will be able to perform over longer periods of time.

Effects of training on cardiac muscle strength

Physical exercise improves the strength and efficiency of the heart muscle by enabling it to circulate more blood while beating less frequently. The contraction of the heart, in effect, becomes more powerful, thus it empties more completely with each beat. As a result, stroke volume (the amount of blood ejected per beat) and cardiac output (the amount of blood ejected per minute) both increase significantly. As exercise training progresses the resting heartbeat slows down, indicating an improvement in the cardiovascular system as a slow heart beat at rest is a major indicator of both a strong heart and good circulation. It is not unusual for a resting pulse rate to be reduced by 15-20 beats per minute as a result of physical training. A resting pulse rate measuring as low as 44 beats per minute has been recorded among marathon runners. Such improvement in the cardiac muscle points to stronger circulation and longer blood flow to reach muscles, tissues, and vital organs. A strong heart ensures adequate supply of oxygen and nutrients to the body. Well developed cardiac muscle recovers quickly after exercise ends as the heart rate, blood pressure, and respiratory rate return to the resting level fairly soon. It should be emphasized that only aerobic exercises such as jogging, cycling, or long-distance swimming can increase the strength of cardiovascular muscle. Short exercises such as short-distance running or weightlifting will have no significant effects on the cardiovascular system.

Effects of various exercises on the cardiovascular system

Both aerobic and anaerobic exercises are used in different sports to varying degrees. The demands they place on the cardiovascular system vary depending on duration and intensity of the activities. Anaerobic contractions, when performed to the maximum, result in a large oxygen debt and a high build up of lactic acid. Such conditions can be observed during sprinting. During an anaerobic activity, such as sprinting, the cardiovascular system cannot meet the oxygen requirements of the muscles. The athlete relies upon oxygen reserves, anaerobic processes, and producing oxygen debt after the exercise ends. Anaerobic exercise increases your ability to respond to emergencies faster; whereas aerobic exercise such as jogging and walking help to lose weight, lower blood pressure, and develop collateral circulation.

During long-duration activities, such as middle distance running and swimming, aerobic metabolism is maximal. The athlete's use of the aerobic process enables him or her to perform over the full duration of a long to middle distance event, reaching maximum levels of oxygen debt only at the end of the race. It is essential to maintain a steady state of oxygen supply during long-duration activities, such as swimming, cycling, running, etc. Only at the beginning and the final segment of a long-distance event should one resort to anaerobic processes. For activities such as tennis, boxing, and football, where a pause in intense activity is followed swiftly by a period of rest or low activity; the problem of oxygen debt repayment is paramount. An athlete who, after intense anaerobic activity, is able to return rapidly toward the resting state has a marked advantage; he can pay back the oxygen debt accumulated during peak efforts. Moreover, such an athlete will be able to produce subsequent peak efforts sooner than a competitor requiring longer to recover from intense anaerobic activity.

One of the major effects of physical activity on the cardiovascular system is an increase in blood circulation to the exercising muscles. Increased circulation is essential because, without it muscular activities cannot be maintained. The increased circulation brings about several benefits:

- It increases the supply of oxygen to the muscles

- It supplies more nutrients and other materials to tissues

- It removes metabolic waste products such as carbon dioxide and lactic acid, which would otherwise accumulate and impair muscular contraction

- It prevents a greater dissipation of heat produced during muscular activities

Cardiovascular changes during exercise

The most important changes occurring during exercise are:

- A higher number of heart beats per minute

- A higher volume of blood ejected with each beat

- An increase in cardiac output

These increases are produced by the direct effects of the nervous and hormonal systems on the heart itself and by a greater return of blood to the heart from the peripheral circulation. Through exercise, the aerobic capacity of the individual increases tremendously. Therefore, he or she is capable of performing an intense level of physical work with little oxygen consumption and with a limited amount of lactic acid accumulation in the blood. Physical training also improves one's capacity for anaerobic work, as a trained person is able to tolerate a higher oxygen debt and a higher accumulation of lactic acid than untrained persons. Therefore, exercise increases one's capacity for both aerobic and anaerobic work.

13

LONG-TERM EFFECTS OF EXERCISE ON THE HEART

This chapter points out the Visible Benefits (muscles get larger) and the Invisible Changes (system improves).

The heart functions like other muscles, deriving its energy from the same chemical reactions. There are, however, some noteworthy differences. They are:

- The activity of the heart never stops

- Unlike other muscles, its oxygen requirement does not increase even during very heavy exercise

- The heart uses lactic acid and pyretic acids for its energy needs

Because of the heart's high level of efficiency, it is reasonable to consider that in a normal subject, the metabolism of the heart itself does not constitute a limiting factor during maximal exercise. Physical activities bring about significant improvements in the respiratory system. Exercise increases the volume of air, oxygen, and carbon dioxide output. About one to two months are needed to bring about a maximum improvement in oxygen and carbon dioxide exchange. For standard workouts, oxygen requirements for the respiratory muscles are reduced. Breathing slows down during rest while the amount of air inspired and expired increases in response to training. Respiratory muscles such as the thoracic, the abdominal, and the diaphragm all become stronger and more effective as a result of training.

Effects of training on aerobic performance

As training progresses, the amount of oxygen supplied to the exercising muscles becomes greater and muscle contraction becomes sufficient to perform higher levels of physical work with little accumulation of lactic acid in the blood. Both the pulse rate and the breathing rate for a standard workload slow down. Individuals are able to do much higher intensity work without incurring oxygen debt. Oxygen debt and lactic acid accumulation occur only at very high levels of intense workout.

Effects of training on anaerobic performance

Physical training increases anaerobic capacity. An individual can tolerate much higher concentration of lactic acid in the blood and a much higher level of oxygen debt as well. A higher accumulation of lactic acid in the blood and a higher oxygen debt are observed in the blood of an athlete who pushes himself to exhaustion. It is believed that a person's determination and motivation probably play an important role in achieving higher anaerobic work, as one must learn to tolerate the discomfort and push oneself to the limit. Through training, an individual learns to endure discomfort, increasing the duration and intensity of exercise as he utilizes his anaerobic capacity.

The level of oxygen consumption is lower during high levels of exercise. The heart rate, respiratory rate, and concentration of lactic acid in the blood, decrease during performance of a steady level of work. Within two or three weeks of training one will reach a new steady level of training. It is possible to increase the workload without oxygen debt.

If training is interrupted for more than one or two months, the efficiency of the workout will be reduced. The pulse rate, respiratory rate, and the concentration of lactic acid in the blood will all be increased. Therefore exercise must be a lifetime program.

Effects of training on the digestive system

When food arrives to the stomach, the involuntary muscles of the stomach wall contract. In some people they contract even when the stomach is partially or entirely empty. The question that has occupied the minds of many for a long time is: How does physical activity affect the digestive system? Furthermore, where does the food first begin to be acted upon by digestive enzymes? The contractions of the stomach following a meal represent digestive peristalsis, which not only involves mixing the gastric contents, but also moving the contents into the duodenums and emptying it. Much investigative work has been done on the effects of various physical activities on the gastric secretions and the frequencies of the emptying of the stomach into the duodenums. All studies show that moderate exercise such as slow walking has a tendency to hasten gastric emptying; whereas exercises such as cycling and running had inhibitory effects on both emptying features and the levels of secretions of enzymes in the stomach wall. Of the four types of gland cells, the chief cells are those that produce pepsin. There is also an oxynitice cell. Its' function is to produce pure hydrochloric acid at the entrance of the stomach. There are gland cells, which secrete alkaline mucus. The function of the mucus cells is to coat the inner lining of the stomach in order to protect it from the action of the hydrochloric acid and pepsin. Gastric juices produced in the stomach in connection with meal taking are controlled by two phases:

- The Reflex Phase—initiates the secretion of gastric juices such as pepsin and hydrochloric acid

- The Second Phase—involves the vegus nerve, the path by which impulses are discharged to the proper gland cells

The impulses are called forth in the act of eating in response to the stimulations of taste, smell, and the overall enjoyment of a meal. A direct correlation exists between the enjoyment of the meal and the secretion of pepsin and hydrochloric acid. The gastric secretions will begin before the act of eating the meal and will continue as long as food remains in the stomach, inhibiting the secretion of gastric juices. The volume of the secretion will not change if exercise precedes the meal.

TOOSHI'S LAW: *"Eating Begins with the Eyes."*

14

FATIGUE AND EXERCISE

TOOSHI'S LAW: "Regular exercise is like honey ... sweetness to the soul; health to the body."

Fatigue is a disturbance in the balance between wear and repair. It is caused by accumulation of lactic acid in the exercising muscles. It may help to understand the degree of fatigue brought about by different physical activities by referring to a concept used in the science of toxicology: the CT. In this concept, the C refers to the concentration of toxic matter and the T refers to the duration of exposure to those toxins. The product, CT, is constant, but as widespread concentration (of a toxin) increases, the duration of exposure (to that toxin) decreases. In exercises such as the 100-meter dash the muscles produce a large amount of lactic acid, too much for athletes to tolerate for a long duration of time, therefore exercise must stop. In long distance running, the athlete may continue running for a long time. In the case of the 100-meter dash, the work is accomplished by reserve oxygen in the blood anaerobically. Moderate, prolonged exercise is done entirely aerobically, utilizing oxygen from outside the body. Under aerobic conditions work is completed through the oxidation of carbohydrates and fats, whereas, under anaerobic conditions work is accomplished solely through oxidation of the body's glucose reserves. On that basis, an outstanding short-distance runner cannot run further than 300 meters at top speed because he rapidly depletes his reserve energy. In moderate exercises very little lactic acid is produced, whereas during strenuous activities a great deal of lactic acid is produced in the muscles, resulting in fatigue.

Physical Stress and Exercise

What is Physical Stress?

Stress constitutes the inability of an individual to adjust him or herself to the demands of the surrounding world with maximum effectiveness and happiness. Stress affects the emotional, social, and mental state of an individual. The term emotion refers to intense feelings with physiological and psychological components. A person does not just experience stress physiologically, but endures certain psychological changes too.

A person who is under stress experiences the following symptoms. Psychological Changes

- Change in sleeping patterns

- Restlessness

- Quick onset of boredom

- Inability to relax

- Decreased desire for recreational activities

- Shorter temper

- Frequent absence from work

- Change in eating patterns

- Lack of sexual desire

- Eating fast

- Talking quickly

- Losing a desire for social interaction/antisocial behavior

Physiological Changes

- Higher pulse rate

- Higher blood pressure

- Lower blood glucose (sugar)

- Higher breathing rate

- Elevated white blood cells

- Lower cardiac output

- Poor circulation

- Slower metabolism

Climate and Exercise

The regulation of body temperature is carried on by physiological mechanisms, which regulate heat loss or gain. In the face of a wide variety of environmental and metabolic temperatures, the internal body temperature is maintained within a relatively narrow range. Several forces affect the internal temperature. These forces come from both within the body and from the outside. One of the most common, acute threats arising within the body is caused by physical exercise. The most common of the external threats are variations in climate. Both internal and external forces impose tremendous strains on two important physiological parameters: firstly, temperature regulation and secondly, the optimal functioning of the cardiovascular system. The balance of heat production and heat loss maintains our body temperature. The body can gain heat internally (from heat produced by metabolism) and externally from heat in the environment. In contrast, the body may lose heat through radiation, convection, conduction, and the evaporation of sweat. The body's major source of heat gain is metabolism. When a person relaxes, his Basal Metabolic Rate (BMR) measures about 70 kilocalories per hour. However, under cold conditions, heat production increases due to contractions of the muscular system (shivering). In hot weather, the body absorbs heat from outside, raising body temperature. Physiologically, exercise can be harmful under hot conditions due to the risk of heat exhaustion. Under such conditions, heat production can exceed thirty times the BMR. The excess heat is produced mainly in the muscles. It is important to realize that blood flowing through the muscles returns directly to the body's core before being circulated to the periphery. When a person exercises heavily, the internal organs are among the first to get the impact of the increased heat production. In hot temperatures, blood circulation is increased to the peripheral regions in order to give off heat and decrease body temperature. This occurs through sweating, whereas in cold temperatures, a large amount of blood moves from the peripheral regions to the internal organs so as to maintain optimal body temperature within a normal range.

Interval training for endurance development

Those who engage in interval training reap tremendous benefits in the development of aerobic and anaerobic performance. Interval training for aerobic development could entail several workloads of slow walking and jogging while maintaining a training pulse rate. This should then be followed by several workloads of higher intensity with pulse rate at 80-90 percent of maximum pulse rate. A person jogging a half-mile with a training pulse rate of 130 then jogs the next half-mile at 160 pulse rate. The individual can repeat this set several times, depending on the training goal. To find training pulse rate and maximum pulse rate use the following formula.

220 - age = Maximum training pulse rate
220 - age = Training pulse rate/100

For a thirty year old person TPR will be [(220 - 30) 70]/100 = 133

15

EXERCISE TRAINING

People who regularly engage in physical activity are able to exert more power, perform physical tasks better, and resist both physical and mental fatigue much better than those who are inactive. Many physiological changes take place as a consequence of regular physical activity. They include:

• Improved neuromuscular coordination

• Increased oxygen supply to the working muscles

• Improved pulmonary ventilation

• Improved oxygen and carbon dioxide exchange with lower energy expenditure by the respiratory muscles

• Increased metabolism and energy production

• Reduced body fat and maintenance of normal healthy body weight

• Slowing of the aging process and increase longevity

What is a Steady State?

The steady state refers to a condition of uniform oxygen consumption. In such a state, exercise may last for a longer period than usual. A steady state is achieved when all the factors regulating a given function are in balance, maintaining at a constant level. When steady state is used in reference to oxygen consumption, it means that oxygen intake equals the oxygen utilized and the body's stores of oxygen remain constant.

Oxygen Debt

Oxygen debt refers to the extent to which the anaerobic process is utilized to perform a workload. When exercise stops, the consumption of oxygen remains at a high level during recovery. The value of the oxygen debt is equal to the amount of oxygen consumed above the resting level from the point at which exercise ceases until the return to the resting level of oxygen consumption; i.e., the point at which recovery is complete. The fact that the oxygen debt has been paid off and that the oxygen consumption has returned to its' resting level does not necessarily imply that the recovery processes are complete. In many instances, heart rate, for example, may remain above the resting level long after oxygen consumption has returned to its resting state.

Body weight affects one's oxygen intake. During aerobic work, oxygen intake varies with the type of exercise performed. In an exercise that involves the movement of the body from one place to another, body weight will play a very important role. The speed at which such exercise is done also plays a significant role in oxygen intake. The skill with which an exercise is performed will effect oxygen consumption. Walking constitutes a good example of the effects of speed and weight on oxygen intake and weight loss.

Mechanical Efficiency

Mechanical efficiency is based on a balance between oxygen intake and oxygen consumption. This balance enables the athlete to continue exercising for longer periods of time. An example is jogging or stationary bicycle riding. But when oxygen consumption goes above oxygen intake, the athlete goes into oxygen dept and fatigue sets in.

Factors affecting oxygen intake during anaerobic work

Anaerobic work refers to exercise under which an individual's oxygen expenditure is at all times in excess of that individual's actual oxygen intake. On that basis, it is not possible to continue such work for a long time.

Physical Fitness

To achieve fitness through exercise, one need not look like Mister Universe or Miss World. What is needed is a normal body weight, enough strength, endurance, and flexibility to meet the demands of daily living faced by all of us.

Physical fitness is divided into four categories with respect to improving the function of the body.

- Muscular strength

- Flexibility

- Cardiovascular endurance

- Muscular endurance

What is Strength?

Muscular strength can be defined as your ability to work against heavy resistance by lifting objects and pushing or pulling heavy objects. The structure and function of these tissues bring tangible, practical benefits giving us the ability to push our stalled cars, carry heavy bags of food, and repair our homes. The muscles empower us to extract ourselves from a variety of difficulties and challenges. Today, mechanical devices have been developed to reduce the need for muscular exertion, bringing affluence to our lifestyles but reducing our physical strength. In order to keep fit in today's world, we must engage in organized, regular exercise. Weight training is an example of an exercise that emphasizes the muscular strength.

What is Flexibility?

Flexibility depends upon the elasticity of the muscles, tendons, and ligaments, as well as the condition of the joints. Flexibility enables the body to move and bend around the joints without pain or difficulty. If flexibility is not maintained, the bones and ligaments will be easily broken and torn.

What is Muscular Endurance?

Muscular endurance refers to the power of the muscles to keep working and exerting force over an extended period of time. Testing muscular endurance would be performing a high number of pull-ups on the bar, doing push-ups, sit-ups, curve, or bench press with more repetitions.

What is Cardiovascular Endurance?

Cardiovascular endurance refers to the ability of the cardiovascular and pulmonary systems to continue pumping blood and oxygen to the working muscles for a long duration. The heart is just like any other muscle; it becomes stronger with physical training such as jogging, cycling, and swimming.

What is Physical Conditioning?

Physical conditioning is required to maintain total fitness. Physical conditioning requires a multitude of adaptations from the body tissues so as to facilitate the work that training demands of them. The safety of an exercise program is the most important consideration for a person beginning physical training. If one is overweight and has not exercised in many years, it is important to have a medical check-up. That medical check-up must include an examination of the following:

- Blood cholesterol

- Blood Pressure

- Blood sugar

- Stress test

How do I begin an exercise program?

If the medical check-up permits, then begin slowly. Gradually build up your strength and endurance. Then slowly and gradually increase your workload. Do not do too much too soon. Keep your long-term goal in mind and have patience. It does not make sense to start with activities that give you pain or leave you with discomfort. Those who start with activities that are beyond their capacity will give up within a very short time. When you work beyond your capacity you break down body tissues. To improve your physical fitness there are two different methods of training:

- **Increase the Frequency.** Increasing the frequency means repeating the activity more often. For example, when using the treadmill you can exercise longer with no increase in speed. When weight training you can increase the repetitions rather than increasing the weight.

- **Increase the Intensity.** Increase the speed of the treadmill while keeping the time of the exercise constant. In weight training routines, increase the weight and keep repetitions constant. You can also use the combination of both. Concerning running, for a few weeks you can increase the time of the run and later the speed of the run. In weight training, work on repetition for a time, then switch to more weight. It all depends on your schedule and objective. If you have less time you may emphasize speed or heavier weights. If you have more time, concentrate on duration and/or repetition.

A Reminder—Bear in mind that physical fitness follows the principle of use and disuse. You will stay in good shape if you keep up your exercise routine on a regular basis. If not, you risk losing your fitness after a short period of inactivity.

Why Warm-Up?

Warm-up exercises play an essential role in the prevention of injury. They protect joints, muscles, ligaments, and cardiac muscle because sudden intense exercise places tremendous stress both upon the heart and upon the muscular structures themselves. By warming-up, the muscles, joints, ligaments and connective tissues are able to endure anything exercise demands of them. A warm-up routine provides a safe transition from a state of rest to physical activity. Remember that temperature, pulse rate, and oxygen intake gradually increase. The body becomes ready for exercise.

Types of Warm-Ups

The type of warm-up exercise you choose depends upon the type of sport you will be engaging in. Nevertheless, there are some effective general warm-up exercises that can be applied to all sports:

- Stretching exercises involving the leg, arm and back muscles

- Slow jogging, for approximately 7-10 minutes is aimed at stimulating circulation and increasing the pulse rate, blood pressure, oxygen intake, as well as body temperature

Why Warm-Down?

Warm-down or cool-down, as it is sometimes called refers to exercises that make a smooth transition from physical activity back to the resting state. More attention should be given to the importance of this transition. The process must be gradual so that both the heart rate as well as the muscles, recuperate slowly. Several minutes of slow jogging or walking will be sufficient in most cases.

Effects of exercise on food intake

A common belief is that engaging in physical exercise stimulates one's appetite. In fact, exercise does not have a major effect on the appetite. Studies have consistently shown that as exercise is increased, it brings about a transition to an active lifestyle from a sedentary one and there is indeed a decrease in caloric intake.

Effects of exercise on obesity

The classification of obesity is based upon the amount of fat that is in the body. A normal man should not be in excess of 15-20 percent body fat and women should not exceed 20-22 percent. It is becoming evident as well that human obesity results in both a marked increase in the number of adipose cells and in cell size. Obesity begins in childhood, in some cases as early as the first year, and leads to a significant increase in the number of fat cells. The number of cells cannot be increased after age nine. At this time fat cell development stops but the size of a fat cell increases as caloric intake increases.

Weight loss is best accomplished through a long-term approach, avoiding the negative effects of a crash diet. It is also advisable to plan a program of progressive exercise in order to compliment the diet. There is some debate over the effectiveness of physical exercise regarding the control of body weight: 3500 calories are needed to metabolize, and lose one pound of body fat. Clearly, dropping a significant amount of body fat is sure to be a long-term process. The point is that weight reduction on a short-term basis through the use of exercise alone is not a successful approach.

The control of body weight through exercise can be achieved only by a proper diet. In the final analysis, weight reduction depends upon achieving a negative caloric balance. That means you must expend more calories than you take in. The most important contributions of exercise are:

- Improve circulation

- Increase metabolism

- Increase the strength of the cardiac muscle

- Reduce emotional stress

- Slow down the aging process

Effects of exercise on quality of life

The human body is designed for physical activity. The heart, lungs, metabolic processes of the body cells all work together to provide energy to sustain physical work. The sustained physical activity of primitive man enabled them to survive. They had to run, climb, jump, and throw. They did these activities to meet the demands of daily life. Today, however, in modern society we do not need to be active to find food or protect ourselves from dangerous animals. We have jobs that require very little physical activity and all modern laborsaving devices at home leaving very little physical work for housewives and our environment does not require that we be physically active. The basic need for physical activity to stimulate the heart, the lungs and metabolic processes remains.

We must inject physical exercise in our daily life to remain fit. But fit for what? We want to be fit in order to perform everyday activities without exercise fatigue. As we become more sedentary, the capacity of the heart and lungs to deliver blood and nutrients to tissues declines, metabolism goes down, blood pressure and blood cholesterol go up, obesity, low back pain, joint disorders and osteoporosis, diabetes and heart disease become the major health problems to deal with. The costs of the treatment of these diseases are beyond capacity of the country to absorb. Today we are consuming more fat, more salt, more sugar, and more food to manage stress.

Problems associated with sedentary living

There was a time in America that the activities of daily living provided plenty of opportunities for physical exercise. These daily activities kept our heart and muscular systems strong. People tended to be fit and obesity was a rarity. The arrival of new technological advances robbed us of our customary activities and left us with today's sedentary lifestyle of comfort. Our typical day begins with rising at 6AM or 7AM, eating a bagel or toaster pastry with coffee from the local drive-up window, working until 5PM and commuting home during rush hour traffic. We arrive home tired and stressed, grabbing a snack or a drink to settle ourselves. Then it's the same routine of eating, watching television and snacking until bedtime. Such is contemporary life for working men and women. Then the weekends provide some social activities including more eating and drinking and driving to get there. A typical social weekend involves more calorie consumption because you are likely faced with appetizers and desserts and very little physical activity.

This seemingly leisurely and sedentary lifestyle has advanced the number of overweight and obese people we see today, many of whom suffer from chronic medical conditions such as hypertension, heart disease, diabetes, and emotional stress. A sedentary lifestyle is not a benign lifestyle; it has prominent side effects on the cardiovascular, respiratory, and muscular systems. For the heart, a lack of physical activity weakens the cardiac muscle and reduces the pumping action (cardiac volume, stroke volume) causing weak circulation. Arteries loose flexibility and become prone to rupture, weakening the vascular system. Circulation slows down, blood pressure goes up, and the chance of suffering a stroke increases. The respiratory muscles weaken, resulting in a reduction in volume (ability to obtain oxygen from the atmosphere), shallow breathing (incomplete expansion of the lungs), and an increased breathing rate, compensating for the lack of oxygen. The decline of these systems continues if you do not alter your sedentary lifestyle. The exchange of oxygen and carbon dioxide lessens giving rise to other respiratory problems such as asthma and infections.

The muscular system responds to overall inactivity by loss of strength, added intramuscular fat, and feeling flabby. The joints, tendons, and ligaments become weak. A weak muscular structure diminishes efficiency and safety of motion and reduces flexibility and equilibrium. The digestive system's speed to digest and eliminate waste material is negatively affected and generally results in constipation. Constipation occurs because there is less oxygen circulating in the body (reduced respiration). There is an overall decline in metabolic functioning leaving you feeling mentally, emotionally, and physically tired. At this stage you may notice a change in your sleeping pattern or have trouble sleeping. By adding physical activity to your daily routine you can start to improve your overall health and well-being.

Exercise and Bone Loss

Lack of exercise produces bone loss. Such a condition is called osteoporosis. It is a disease in which the bones lose calcium. The bones become thin, brittle and breakable. Osteoporosis is a major problem in the United States affecting 25 million people. It causes millions of fractures among people age 45 and over. The major cause of osteoporosis is not lack of calcium in the body; it is lack of exercise, which prevents calcium from being metabolized. We all heard about the first group of astronauts, who came back from space with lost bone density. That was the reason for putting a stationary bicycle in the spacecraft for astronauts to exercise while they were in space.

Exercise and Stress

In our fast pace of living, many changes take place in our modern world. People are unable to cope with stress, resulting heart disease, ulcers, and many other health-related problems. It is believed that physical exercise can serve as an outlet for the release of the stress and provide a relaxation to the nervous system. Exercise makes people better prepared to deal with stress. Today, more and more medical authorities are encouraging people to use physical exercise as an important method in treating depression.

Stress is caused by disturbance of homeostatic balance. Both physiological and psychological conditions can promote stress. The reaction of the nervous system to emotional and physiological conditions is exactly identical. But not everybody reacts to stress the same way. Some people function better under stress than others. The differences in the reactions of people to emotional crises are due to various ways in which they perceive stress. Some magnify the importance of an event, whereas others consider it not to be important.

Physiological changes of stress

Environmental forces are constantly bombarding our bodies. Some of these forces produce pleasant experiences. Others cause fear, anger or rage, which stimulate the secretion of hormones. Hormones such as epinephrine or norepinephrine are produced when the body becomes stressed.

Stress causes the following changes in the body:

- Heart rate and stroke volume increase

- Blood vessels in the skin, kidney and internal organs become constricted, decreasing blood flow to these organs

- Systolic blood pressure increases

- Secretion of the digestive glands and blood flow is decreased

- Blood glucose is increased

- Rate of ventilation goes up

- Muscle tension is increased

- Increased metabolism of working muscles

Emotional conflicts brought on by the turmoil in our present society stimulate our glands, which prepares the body for a stressful experience. Modern societies, however, make relief of tension within the body virtually impossible. People are not provided with techniques to deal with such problems. Only physical exercise can neutralize hormone secretion and reduce stress.

16

EXERCISE WORK OUT

How often to exercise

Studies show that fewer than three workouts per week appear to be insufficient to produce measurable cardiovascular benefits. Three workouts per week have been demonstrated to be beneficial for most sedentary people. After a moderate level of training has been achieved, the frequency should be increased to four to five workouts per week.

How long to exercise

An average exercise session should be at least 30 minutes in duration with 5 to 10 minutes warm up and 5 to 10 minutes cool down.

How hard to exercise

The intensity of exercise is probably the most important part of an exercise program. It has been already established that the threshold necessary to produce measurable gain in cardiovascular training must be 70 percent of maximum pulse rate. The aerobic exercise will not produce any desirable benefit if it is below seventy percent maximum training pulse rate.

One of the most frequent mistakes made by those who are beginning an exercise program is to work too hard too soon. The resultant general and localized muscular soreness experienced by formerly sedentary people is often a turning off rather than a turning on to exercise.

People over 35 years of age who want to begin an aerobic exercise program should have a medical examination to make sure that they are safe to exercise. The medical examination should include:

- Blood pressure

- EKG

- Blood glucose

- Blood cholesterol

- Stress test

Exercise and Aging

The guidelines used in exercise are the same for men, women and older people. Recommendations:

- Exercise should be avoided when a person is ill. Exercise can aggravate minor illnesses.

- Exercise should be avoided in very hot and cold environments

- Exercise should be avoided after eating a heavy meal

- Sauna baths, steam rooms, and hot showers should be avoided immediately after exercise. These activities, which dilate blood vessels in skin and divert blood from internal organ to the surface of the body, may cause dizziness, high blood pressure and low blood circulation in the heart. It may cause a heart attack.

Aging and sedentary living have a predictable effect on the human body that results in a gradual decline in the functional capacity of:

- Cardiovascular system

- Pulmonary system

- Physical strength

- Blood pressure

- Increased body fat

- Flexibility

The deteriorations do not have to be accepted as a natural consequence of aging or the inevitable. It is a known fact that much of the decline in functional capacity is more the result of a sedentary life style than aging. Evidence shows that every one of the changes listed can be reversed or at least have the rate of progression slowed down by proper exercise.

Exercise related injuries

We must be aware that exercise may cause injuries that range from minor to serious. Those without prior experience in exercise must follow some rules:

- Before committing to an exercise regimen have a medical examination

- Start exercise slowly and gradually progress. Keep speed and duration low.

- If you are walking or jogging, find a safe place so that you do not run into trouble. Avoid highways, streets and high traffic areas. Parks are an excellent place to exercise.

- Get adequate warm up before exercise so that you do not get pulled muscles or cause cramps

- Wear suitable clothing and shoes according to the weather

Muscle Soreness

Muscle pain or soreness usually occurs after high intensity exercise. Some people get stiffness in the muscles. Others feel pain after heavy and intensive exercise. It is due to the accumulation of metabolic products such as lactic acid. Such pain subsides shortly after the intensity of exercise is reduced. Muscular soreness that follows unaccustomed exercise usually occurs within two days and then gradually subsides after another two or three days. This kind of soreness is due to overstretching the muscles' elastic components. Muscle spasms and muscle cramps result from the lack of calcium and magnesium in the muscles. The recovery from muscle soreness can be enhanced by warm compresses or a warm bath, accompanied by light exercise, which prevents adhesions during the healing process.

17

WOMEN AND EXERCISE

TOOSHI'S LAW: *"Nature is very cruel."*
The same hormones that give shapeliness and softness give menstrual pain and
symptoms of menopause

In recent years the number of women participating in aerobic exercise has been increasing tremendously because they are more aware of the impact of exercise on their overall health and well being. All studies show that women's response to exercise is not much different than men's. There are only a few exceptions.

Iron Deficiency.

Because of the menstrual cycle, women lose iron. Prolonged, regular exercise tends to produce an iron-related blood disorder, namely anemia. Iron deficiency causes weakness and fatigue. Vitamin C must be taken in order to increase the absorption of iron.

Menstrual Cycle.

The onset of the menstrual cycle is different among women as is the degrees of discomfort, lack of energy, pain around abdomen, constipation, sleep disorders, and mood changes associated with menstrual cycle. Evidence suggests that severe, prolonged exercise such as jogging and swimming is associated with the cessation of menstruation. The cycle returns to normal when training becomes less intense. During these few days it is advisable for women not to engage in intense exercise. During menstrual cycle loss of body fat among women who exercise very hard may reduce estrogen production. Presence of estrogen is an important condition for normal menstrual cycle as well as the deposition of minerals in the female bones. Exercising during the menstrual cycle can stabilize hormones and increase oxygen in the blood, whereby relaxing the body, reducing abdominal pain and feelings of depression and fatigue. Thirty minutes a day of aerobic exercise is recommended to alleviate most symptoms commonly associated with menstruation.

Exercise during pregnancy.

A healthy and physically fit woman feels better during pregnancy and delivery is easier than one who is unfit. Evidence from animal studies plus what is known about the human response to exercise and training raises questions about exercising during pregnancy. High intensity of exercise increases heat production and may have negative effect on the health of the fetus.

Physical exercise during pregnancy may cause the following problems:

- Oxygen deprivation of the fetus

- Production of high temperature

- Inadequate nutrition

- Metabolic alteration

- Change in hormone production

During exercise, the body diverts blood from the kidney, abdominal organs, stomach, intestine, and liver to the exercising muscles and skin for providing energy, and cooling the blood circulation and oxygen delivery to uterus is sharply reduced. This reduction of blood circulation and oxygen may cause a severe injury to the fetus. Excessive body temperature during long and hard exercise may produce birth defects and in later pregnancy can induce premature labor. Women who exercise during pregnancy should monitor their body temperature at the conclusion of each session and not allow the temperature to exceed 101 F. Effort should be made to cool down immediately. There is no reason for a healthy woman not to exercise; in fact she should take thirty minutes daily for walking to stimulate circulation.

Pregnant women should benefit from the following plan.

- Women who have been previously sedentary should not undertake a strenuous exercise program

- Women who are already training hard should reduce the intensity

- Pregnant women should avoid exercising for long periods of time. Doing hard exercise may produce dehydration that should be avoided.

Change in body weight

Most people expect a dramatic weight loss when they embark on an exercise program. Well, I hate to disappoint you but unless you are quite overweight, there will be little, if any, reduction in total body weight. In fact you may gain weight. Remember muscle is much heavier than fat; as the fat is exercised away from inside the muscle, total muscle mass will increase and it is likely you may gain some weight about 2 to 3 pounds. Remember this happens if you are not overweight. What happens to muscle when it is exercised naturally? All muscles are long and lean with very little fat. Then as we get older and more out of shape, fat slowly invades the muscle. The shape of muscle becomes short and squat. The muscle eventually becomes so saturated with fat that it cannot hold anymore and then the fat begins to accumulate outside that short and squat muscle. When your diet has little effect on the fat inside muscle and nothing happens to the muscle shape, it is still short and squat. When you exercise, exercise removes intramuscular fat away and the muscle returns to its original shape; long and lean. Loss of subcutaneous fat under the skin will result in change of body size but usually the person's shape merely seems to be a smaller version of what it was before the loss.

Spot Reduction

Since fat concentrates in specific areas of the body, most people feel that they must super exercise those areas to get rid of fat. Women are concerned with the deposit on the hips and thighs and men worry about the fat around the midsection and so they join health spas that guarantee to remove fat from specific areas or they buy all kinds of pulling, punching, rolling devices to jiggle away that fat. There are two favorite modes of spot reduction:

- Passive

- Active

Neither of these works! In fact there is no known technique, short of surgery, for removing fat from any particular place in the body. Passive spot reduction includes the pulley and bull rollers often found in health spas. The theory is that if you beat it long enough you are bound to break up the fat and disburse it. It is also foolish to lose weight in a sauna or steam bath. These are simply very danger-ous. These methods can lead to dehydration. Dehydration may drop your blood pressure to a level that causes dizziness or heart attack.

The active method of spot reduction is involved using the muscle that is directly beneath the fat deposit. It is like trying to get rid of the fat on your belly by trying to do sit ups. No matter how many sit ups you do a day you are not going to reduce the fat, but what sit-ups will do is to build the muscles under your abdomen. Abdominal fat must be thought of as belonging to the whole body. In women, subcutaneous fat is deposited first at the back of the thigh, then on the outside of the thigh, then the hips and finally in the upper body. If you are a woman with fat in those places and you start a daily bicycle exercise program, the fat will decrease in reverse order from the way it was deposited even though bicycle is a leg exercise. You will lose fat from your arms first and your legs last.

The puckering in woman's legs, often called cellulite is just lots of fat under a slightly different skin texture. But I have to remind you that you cannot get rid of that no matter what type of exercise or manipulation is used in that spot. You will not get rid of it. But if you exercise your whole body, especially aerobic exercises you will trim down all over.

Weight Training

As previously discussed, exercising isolated muscles in the body will do little to decrease the fat around those muscles. Fat deposits are only decreased with aero-bic (whole body) exercise. However, weight-training exercises are good for improving strength. A person can increase the size and strength of specific mus-cles; for example, skiers can improve the strength of their legs doing squats with barbells on their shoulders. The pectoralis muscles across the front of the chest can be enlarged through bench pressing. These muscles support the breasts, giv-ing women a change in their figures. Weight training also helps to gain weight. Even push-ups, sit-ups and chin-ups are considered to be good weight training. In weight training you do not utilize fat from any part of the body. The calories used here come from glucose rather than fat calories. Those who want to improve their physical fitness must do aerobic exercise for weight control and weight training for strength.

Exercise and Weight Loss

We use very few calories during any aerobic exercise such as jogging, cycling or swimming. Consequently, you cannot lose very much weight through exercise.

However, exercising makes a significant contribution to our total health in the following ways:

- Metabolism. Metabolism of the tissues generates more heat and extra energy to the body and increases burning of the fat.

- Circulation. The tissues receive more blood and exchange carbon dioxide and oxygen quickly. The metabolism of nutrients speeds up.

- Reducing mental stress. When your mind is occupied with exercise external forces have limited effect on your nervous system. This process takes tension out of your nervous system and relaxes your whole, entire body.

- Slows down the aging process

- Increases self-confidence and self-image

18

SELECTION OF AEROBIC EXERCISE

Most anxiously wrestle with overweight and boredom. In this chapter, I describe how you can select the right exercise program to meet your physical and emotional needs. Boredom comes from lack of knowledge when you do not understand the value exercise has on the heart, blood pressure, cholesterol, and mental health. Once you understand the value of exercise, the boredom goes away. That's why some people are "addicted to exercise."

Exercise should give you not only physical benefit; it also should give pleasure of doing it. Many people comment that they get bored doing the same exercise day after day. The reason for complaining is that they select aerobic exercise, which is not suitable to them. Adapt exercise to what fits your way of life, your job, your schedule and your physical fitness level. Start exercise slowly with lower pulse rate and increase it as you progress. Many people fail because they:

- Choose the wrong exercise

- Exercise too hard at the beginning with no regard to pulse rate. You should select exercise that gives you correct pulse rate and add more strenuous exercise later.

Types of aerobic exercises

The following are aerobic exercises. You can choose any of them that are suited for you.

Jogging and Running

The most well known aerobic exercise is a jogging and running program. It is easy to start and the only equipment required is a pair of good shoes. A jogger should try to run as flat-footed as possible to avoid shin splints, jogger's heel, pulled Achilles' tendons and strained calf muscles. If you are over thirty, I recommend taking a stress test to see if your heart is in good condition.

Walking

Walking is an excellent exercise for all ages. This is excellent exercise for older people since it is not traumatic to the knee and joints as is jogging. Just be sure the walk is brisk enough to maintain your heart rate over 120 pulse beats per minute in order to get your cardiovascular system working.

Swimming

Swimming can improve your heart and your lungs. It is an excellent aerobic exercise. It is also good exercise for limbering up all the muscles in the arms and legs. In swimming as in jogging you need to swim at least 30 minutes a day, non-stop. You start slowly and build up your endurance gradually but progressively. You may select both jogging and swimming for your aerobic workout, depending on the suitability of weather, or place you can use for jogging or swimming.

Cross Country Skiing

This is the most intense aerobic exercise. Cross-country skiing gives all the benefits of running or walking without any of their bad effects. Instead of pounding your feet on a hard surface you glide along smoothly. In addition, you use your arms a lot more to help move your body.

Cycling

This is an excellent aerobic exercise for overweight or older people. Those with back problems prefer this exercise. In fact, cycling in general seems to eliminate the problems that constantly plague runners such as pulled muscles, twisted joints, and sore tendons. Both stationary bikes and outdoor bikes have the same aerobic benefits. In both types of cycling, the exercise pulse rate tends to be the same (your training pulse rate).

Stationary Bicycle

This is very good exercise for older, unfit and overweight people. You should plan to buy a reasonably good bike that can last longer. Stay away from motor driven models. Also avoid the elliptical machine that calls for moving your arms while peddling. I recommend stationary models made by Monarch or Schwinn.

HOW TO USE THE STATIONARY BIKE—simply adjust the tension or the speed until you reach your training pulse rate. If you want to slim down your thighs, keep the tension down and pedal faster.

Rowing Machine

The rowing machine is the best aerobic exercise. A good rowing machine exercises all the major muscles in the body: the arms, back and abdomen. Make sure to get one with a seat that slides so that you can push with your legs. When you are exercising with a rowing machine make sure that you do not go beyond your training pulse rate.

Treadmill

Fast walking on a treadmill is comparable to moderate jogging. Exercising with a treadmill prevents you from developing sore knees or back associated with jogging. You can adjust the speed of the treadmill according to your level of physical fitness. If you are a beginner you should start with walking for several weeks until you will be able to exercise for 30 minutes without stopping. Then you can increase your speed. Eventually you will be able to jog. Remember to always pay attention to your training pulse rate and not go beyond it.

Running in Place

This is an excellent indoor exercise because all age groups can use it. Each person can adjust the pace according to that individual's level of fitness. Running in place must be performed on a soft mat. The speed of running in place should raise your pulse to the level of your exercise-training rate.

Chair Step Exercise

This exercise is a very good exercise for the heart and lungs. It improves your cardiovascular system and strengthens leg muscles. It is very easy to do. Just follow this rhythm, up-up, down-down. This exercise is very good for trimming thighs and calf muscles.

Recovery of pulse rate

Pulse rate after exercise is one of the best ways to evaluate the condition of the heart. It is an important health indicator. Pulse rate drops after exercise. At first there is a sharp drop and than it levels off and gradually drops to the resting level. The time it takes for the heart to recover all the way down to the resting heart rate is not significant. The critical period of recovery is in the first minute after exercise.

How to calculate your recovery pulse rate

Take your pulse for six seconds immediately at the end of an exercise and then again one minute later. Subtract the second number from the first and divide by ten as you see in the formula below.

$$\frac{\text{Exercise Pulse - 1-Minute Pulse}}{10} = \text{Recovery Pulse}$$

If you get a high number it means your heart recovers quickly and indicates a healthy heart. Example: If your exercise pulse is 140 and your one-minute after exercise pulse is 100 then divided by 10 it will give you a recovery of 4. If you look at the recovery table below, you find "4" on the recovery table is very good.

Recovery Table

Less than 2 Poor	
2-3	Fair
3-4	Good
4-6	Excellent
More than 6	Superior

To be physically fit, we must train our muscular and cardiovascular systems. The strength and vitality of these systems decline very rapidly after the age of forty. Therefore training of these two systems must be started before age 30 or better yet during high school.

Cardiovascular Exercise

The best exercises to help improve the cardiovascular system are:

- Walking

- Jogging

- Stationary Bicycle

- Swimming

- Hiking

- Cross country skiing

If you have no experience and you want to begin exercise you should follow this program:

Step One—Walk

> At the beginning of an exercise program you should walk with a slower pace like you are walking at the mall. Do not let your pulse go over 130 beats per minute.
>
> A walking program should follow this pattern:
>
> Walk 15 minutes
>
> Rest 2 minutes
>
> Repeat three times

Follow this program for two weeks. Then each two weeks add another five minutes to your program until you walk thirty minutes non-stop. After you reach thirty minutes gradually increase your speed but be sure that your pulse does not go beyond 130 beats per minute.

Step Two—Jog

> If you have experience in jogging but have been sedentary, you should start walking first for at least two weeks. After two weeks, begin jogging thirty minutes per day and add thirty minutes of weight training per day. This schedule should be practiced at least three times per week. Never let your pulse go beyond 130 beats per minute.

Always begin your exercise first with a cardiovascular exercise (walking or jogging), and then do weight training. Do not begin your program with weight training first because it is important to warm-up your joints, muscles, and tendons to prevent injury and to gradually increase your body temperature to prevent injury and to gradually increase your body temperature to prepare for a safe weight training session. Always be aware to weight train with a partner or in the company of a trainer, never alone.

With every passing year, the pounds seem to creep on. Muscles become weak and strength goes down. Starting at around age thirty Americans gain about a pound a year. By the age of fifty they may be carrying an extra 20 pounds of weight and facing such problems as heart disease, diabetes and high blood pressure. At first glance, the cause is simple arithmetic. We eat more calories than we expend. Starting at the age of thirty you begin to lose muscle tissue, the body's main calorie burner, and it is replaced by fat. Muscle burns three times as many calories as fat, even at rest.

Exercise and Muscle Mass

Weight training exercise fights the loss of muscle mass and increases muscle tissue and also strengthens bones, ligaments, which helps you stay active longer and healthier. On that basis I have planned a special weight-training program in conjunction with cardiovascular exercise. It is very important that you follow this program three times a week for one hour each session

Dr. Tooshi's exercise program is made up from:

- Weight Training Exercise

- Cardiovascular Exercise

Weight Training Program

There are two types of weight training programs. One promotes circulation and definition to muscles, whereas the other increases the bulk and strength of the muscles. To increase blood circulation to the muscle athletes should use lighter weights and more repetitions.

To increase muscle size athletes should use heavier weights with less repetition.

	Increase Circulation		Increase Strength	
Station	Reps	Sets	Reps	Sets
Bench Press	15	3	6	3
Leg Press	15	3	6	3
Curl	15	3	6	3
Lats	15	3	6	3
Sit-up	30	3	30	3
Military Press	15	3	6	3

For safety reasons never exercise alone in the gym.

19

DR. TOOSHI'S EXERCISE PROGRAM

The secret of stretching longevity and maintaining a youthful appearance is linked to your degree of physical activity. People who live longer without chronic disease are typically more active individuals. It appears that regular daily exercise and activity is a miracle treatment for the body and soul. Exercise also helps energize the body, reduce depression, maintain youthful appearance and reduce susceptibility to chronic disease. Exercise stimulates the brain to produce endorphins. Endorphins create good feelings, cheerfulness, and positive self-image. However, inactivity typically causes poor circulation, fatigue, depression, and poor self-image. Inactivity also leads to accelerating the aging process and weakening the immune system.

The most important benefit of exercise is physical fitness. Physical fitness has two components:

- Cardiovascular fitness

- Muscular fitness

The goals of cardiovascular fitness are:

- Increase the pumping action of the heart so that more blood can be delivered to the tissues

- Increase oxygen supply to the tissues

- Increase efficiency of the lungs

- Control blood pressure

- Improve the metabolism of the body

- Develop collateral circulation

The goals of muscular fitness are:

- Increase the strength of muscles

- Increase endurance of the muscles

- Prevent a decline of muscular strength caused by aging

Cardiovascular and strength fitness require two different forms of exercise. Cardiovascular fitness is achieved by endurance exercises such as:

- Walking

- Jogging

- Stationary Bicycle

- Swimming

Muscular fitness is achieved only by weight training or resistance activities, such as pulling or pushing a heavy load. One should participate in both cardiovascular and endurance fitness on a regular basis. A work out session should be divided into two segments. Sixty percent of the time should be used for cardiovascular activities and forty percent for a weight-training program. Before participating in a physical fitness program both men and women over 35 years of age must have a physical. The physical must include:

- Stress test

- Blood pressure

- Blood sugar

- Cholesterol

Exercise Pulse Rate

To participate in cardiovascular exercise, one must find exercise pulse rate. To find one's exercise pulse rate use the following formula:

Exercise Pulse Rate (TPR) = $\dfrac{(220 - Age) \times 70}{100}$ =

To find the proper speed for walking, running or cycling one should exercise at any speed for five minutes and then stop, quickly take the pulse rate for 10 seconds and then multiply by six. That gives you your pulse rate for one minute. If that pulse is less than your exercise (TPR) rate, then increase your speed. If the pulse rate is more than your exercise pulse, then reduce your speed.

Muscular Fitness

There are seven major weight exercises that can improve your muscular strength. They are:

- Bench press

- Curl

- Military press

- Leg press

- Lats

- Dead lift

- Sit-ups

To determine how much weight to begin with, select a weight, and test if you can lift it comfortably six times. That should be the weight at which to start each of your exercises. As you progress, you can increase either the weight or the repetitions.

You have options:

If you want to improve the size of your muscles, increase the weight and keep the repetitions the same. If you want to improve endurance and circulation as well as definition of your muscles you should increase repetitions and keep the same weight. Each weight exercise should be done with six repetitions and three sets each to increase muscle definition. When you begin exercising, it is best to follow the sequence above. Do not change the order.

Cardiovascular Fitness

If you have been inactive for some time, you should follow this modified program:

- Jog on the treadmill or outdoors for five minutes and rest two minutes. Repeat six times.

- After two weeks, jog seven and one-half minutes and rest two minutes. Repeat three times.

- Add five minutes to your running every two weeks until you can jog or walk forty minutes straight.

You must remember that you must monitor your exercise pulse rate at all times. If you go beyond your exercise pulse rate, your lungs will not obtain adequate oxygen to meet the demand of your body and your cardiovascular system will go into oxygen debt. Exercising below your exercise pulse rate will prevent you from getting cardiovascular benefits from your efforts.

Cardiovascular Exercise Program

Jog or Walk		Rest	Repetitions
Week/Cycle			
I	5 minutes	2	6
II	7.5 minutes	2	4
III	10 minutes	2	3
IV	15 minutes	2	2
V	20 minutes	2	2
VI	30 minutes	2	1
VII	35 minutes	2	1
VIII	40 minutes	2	1

By the end of the above regimen you will be physically fit. Your training pulse will drop. You may increase your speed or increase your time. It is the same as with weight training. As your training continues, you can increase the amount of weight or repetitions.

Diabetes and Exercise

There are two types of diabetes: Type I and Type II. Type I is hereditary and begins in childhood. Type II occurs in adulthood and is caused by excessive consumption of carbohydrates. Diabetes is one of the most dangerous diseases of mankind. It causes blood clotting, blindness and kidney failure. Diabetes is caused by consumption of high carbohydrate foods, especially starches, sugar, cake, pie, muffins, candy and soft drinks. These foods raise the blood sugar and stimulate the secretion of insulin from the pancreas. Consumption of these foods on a regular basis causes the pancreas to become overworked, and eventually stop producing insulin. Blood sugar builds up in the blood and causes high blood sugar. Since the body no longer uses sugar, the excess sugar shows up in the urine.

There are two ways you can lower blood sugar:

• Lowering the consumption of carbohydrates

• Regular daily exercise, especially cardiovascular exercise such as walking or jogging

Exercise utilizes sugar as fuel for the body. Physical exercise helps to open up pores of cells, allowing the blood sugar to enter the cells. Sugar inside the cells combines with oxygen to produce energy for physical activities. Through exercise along with consuming low carbohydrate foods, the blood sugar can be controlled without medication. Use of low glycemic foods such as fruits, vegetables, whole wheat and rye breads are essential for people with diabetes.

Glycemic Index

Carbohydrate foods such as fruits and vegetables and whole grains have a glycemic index less than eighty. These foods do not cause an increase in blood sugar as much as starches do. But foods with a glycemic index over eighty will increase blood sugar. Foods with a glycemic index over eighty are sugar, soft drinks, candy, pie, white bread, muffins, pasta, rice and potatoes.

Physiology of weight loss

All tissues of the body require fuel for a variety of activities. The fuel the body needs comes from the foods we consume. We consume food from sources such as carbohydrates, proteins and fats. The vitamins and minerals we require provide assistance for digestion and metabolism of foods in order to be used efficiently. Among all the foods we eat, the body first selects carbohydrate foods before it utilizes the fats we consume. No fat or protein can be metabolized for energy production if we eat a diet rich in carbohydrate foods. Fats will only be used for energy if the level of carbohydrate in the diet is reduced. Only then will fats and proteins enter the metabolic process. Accordingly if you want to lose weight, you must lower the level of carbohydrate food in the diet. A high carbohydrate diet will not help you to lose weight no matter how much exercise you do.

Performance activities are divided into three categories:

- Electrical activity of the nervous system such as thinking, hearing, feeling and awareness of the environment

- Mechanical energy or the bodily activities of daily life such as walking, running, lifting, writing, and eating

- Basal Metabolic Rate or internal activities such as the activities of the heart, lungs, kidneys, and digestive system

Each of these activities requires energy. This energy comes from carbohydrate foods. The calories utilized for these activities are called basal metabolic consumption. To reduce body weight, people should:

- Reduce the portion size of food they consume to help shrink the stomach and reduce appetite

- Select foods containing less fat, especially animal fat

- Reduce the number of snacks, especially those that have high fat, high sugar and salt. Eat fruit instead.

- Reduce carbohydrate consumption, especially noncomplex carbohydrates such as cake, cookies, ice cream, etc

- Engage in aerobic exercises but not weight training. Weight training utilizes very little energy and has no positive effect on the cardiovascular system.

20

EXERCISE AND MENTAL STRESS

What is Mental Stress?

We are able to process information about the world we live in through our primitive nervous system. When we receive stimuli that are stressful, our nervous system reacts like an army responding to a battle call. The call to battle or warning alarm is located in the hypothalamus gland within the brain. The hypothalamus triggers a series of reactions to cope with a dangerous or difficult situation. A number of things happen concerning your level of energy and alertness. Through the sympathetic nervous system the adrenal gland receives a signal and is stimulated. It responds by pouring two hormones, epinephrine and nor epinephrine into the bloodstream. An increase in these hormones triggers a rise in the secretion of insulin and thyroxin, from the pancreas and thyroid gland respectively. A rise in insulin and thyroxin speeds up the metabolism of sugar and our energy level increases making us ready for a" fight or flight" response. Our heartbeat and pulse increase, blood pressure rises, and blood flow transfers to the larger muscles in the body making us ready to fight or run. The trouble is that modern stressors or problems cannot be solved with primitive responses or in physical ways. We cannot fight our bosses or run away from our jobs and responsibilities. Our bodies are now in a state of alert but with no way to physically discharge the excess energy without jeopardizing our livelihoods or relationships. Being alert in this manner is termed as being in a state of arousal or tension. Tense people are generally not efficient and not equipped to recognize that their coping patterns cause more problems than they solve. Failure to cope with unresolved tension leads to anxiety and depression. High levels of blood sugar that we cannot utilize only contribute to our anxieties and no longer serve the original fight or flight function effectively.

When we are feeling bad, our brains secrete a chemical called cortisone. Cortisone may interfere with insulin sensitivity and is often elevated in depressed people. Cortisone may also make depressed people more prone to osteoporosis because cortisone appears to interfere with the ability of bones to absorb calcium. Pre-menopausal women who are depressed have a much higher rate of bone loss than their non-depressed counterparts. This disparity increases as women pass through menopause. Depression contributes to the high occurrence of women getting osteoporosis. Another class of chemicals, the pro-inflammatory cytokines has been implicated in osteoporosis and diabetes, but their role is less clear.

Links between depression and other diseases including cancer, Parkinson's disease, epilepsy, stroke, and Alzheimer's disease have been identified. In some cases researchers have clues, if not definitive evidence, as to which molecules might be involved. In Parkinson's disease, the problem is the death of cells in the brain that produce the neurotransmitter dopamine. While dopamine is crucial to the control of movement it is probably a major factor in mood (i.e. depression) as well. Depression almost certainly has multiple causes that produce similar symptoms.

What we experience as feelings or good or bad are at the cellular level and are no more than a complex interaction of chemicals and electrical activity. Depression represents an imbalance in that interaction, one that can kill just as directly and more objectively than physical ailments. Each year in the United States an estimated 30,000 people commit suicide, with the vast majority of cases attributable to depression. But depression's physical toll goes far beyond the number of people who take their own life and even beyond the impact on the relationships and productivity of depressed individuals. The effects of depression cost the US economy some fifty billion dollars a year.

Symptoms of Depression

- Feelings or restlessness, tapping or pacing

- Changes in heart beat, hard and irregular

- Muscular tightness and tenseness

- Shallow and rapid breathing

- Dry mouth

- Feeling tired or easily fatigued

- Backache

- Headache

- Tenseness in shoulder, neck and back muscles

- Teary and watery eyes

- Bloated stomach

- Feeling heavy and unfit

- Eating fast

- Talking fast

- No desire for sex

- Lack of involvement with people

How to relieve stress

- Regular exercise

- Listening to music

- Hot bath

- Yoga

- Reducing sweets and starchy foods in the diet

- Losing weight

- Increasing fruits, vegetables, and sea foods in the diet

- Praying

- Meditation

- Cutting down on salt intake

- Avoiding being alone

- Avoiding associating with unhappy people

- Reading or writing about a subject you enjoy

- Staying away from bad news or sad movies

Some people experience mood swings and turn to forms or self-medication to relieve their symptoms. It is true that illegal drugs and prescription drugs may produce pleasure and relax the body, but the effects of drugs are temporary. In a short time the effect of these drugs fades away and leaves a permanent scar. The user experiences hopeless feelings and becomes psychologically disabled. One of the best ways to get rid of stress is regular daily exercise and meditation. Exercise gives you personal satisfaction, a good self-image, and mental energy. Daily exercise produces a chemical in the brain that gives pleasure, vitality, and high spirits naturally. Self-confidence and self-realization resurface with daily regular exercise. Physical exercise also provides an outlet to reduce stress and aggravation associated with daily life. Exercise improves your cardiovascular system, circulation, and metabolism. Exercise also plays a role in weight loss, job performance, and helps one sleep better. A physically fit person lives longer, performs daily activities more efficiently, and participates more fully in life events than those who are inactive and use drugs to reduce stress.

Mental Stress

Stress is a major health problem in America. It is the most dangerous medical problem among white-collar workers. It is responsible for cancer, stroke, high blood pressure, digestive disorders and heart attacks. Stress is part of life; it has been genetically imbedded in us by nature to promote life. Usually, stress is very high among intelligent people who see the world clearly and can detect problems better.

Then the questions that should be raised are:

- What is stress?

- What causes stress?

At rest when the body is at peace by itself, all parts of the body including the heart, lungs, kidneys, liver, and digestive system work together in harmony and get along with each other very well. All vital signs, pulse, blood pressure and temperature are within normal range. A person has a lot of energy, feels good, and sleeps well. But when outside agents or forces threaten the body, its peaceful environment and working harmony of systems are disturbed and begin to break down. As soon as the body detects a threat, the body's defense system begins to mobilize to respond to the threat. One of the most powerful defense agents in the body is a hormone called epinephrine. This hormone is produced by the adrenal glands, which are located on top of the kidneys. Epinephrine helps to generate energy to the body to fight and overcome a threat.

- Epinephrine stimulates the liver and the liver converts the stored energy glycogen to glucose and sends it throughout the body via the circulatory system

- Epinephrine stimulates the heart, increases pulse rate and blood pressure, and speeds up circulation in order to deliver energy to the muscles to fight or flee

In the primitive world when man was faced with danger, he had two choices to defend himself. He could fight or run away. In both cases, the muscles of primitive man used the energy built up in the muscle. After he escaped danger, his body returned to a resting state. His body relaxed and his system began to work in harmony again. Yet in our modern society we cannot defend ourselves by fighting or running away. Primitive man's methods do not work for us. For example, if we face problems in our job, we cannot physically fight with our bosses or run away from our jobs. We stay and take the punishment. The body though remains in a fighting state with elevated blood sugar, high pulse rate and blood pressure. If such a state continues, anxiety and frustration build up. That anxiety and frustration is responsible for the development of cancer, heart attacks, diabetes, stroke, acid reflux, constipation, difficulty sleeping, and low energy.

As long as high blood sugar, high blood pressure, and high pulse rate stay with us, frustration and anxiety will continue to rise. Now, an alternative can overcome this problem, namely regular physical exercise. Research shows that during physical exercise, blood sugar is used, blood pressure and pulse return to resting level, and all parts of the body begin to work together again. Thirty to forty minutes daily of cardiovascular exercise is the most important remedy for prevention of anxiety and depression.

Symptoms of depression and anxiety

Physiological Symptoms

- High blood pressure

- High pulse rate

- High blood sugar

- Acid reflux

- Constipation

Psychological Symptoms

- Insomnia

- Headache

- Lack of energy

- Mood changes

- Anger

- Restlessness

- Lack of sexual desire

- Feeling tired

- Losing patience

I am not saying that regular exercise is a solution to all your problems. What physical exercise will do is to prevent succumbing to the dangerous effects and outcomes of mental stress.

PART IV

TECHNICAL DISCUSSIONS

21

YOUR CIRCULATORY SYSTEM

This chapter deals with the function of the heart, vascular system, stroke volume, cardiac output, and blood pressure.

The Vascular System

The primary function of the circulatory system is the transportation of food and oxygen to the body's cells and, in this sense, that capacity plays a vital role in cellular metabolism. The circulatory system also transports water and electrolytes, making an important contribution to the maintenance of fluid volume and pH levels, as well as control of body temperature. Moreover, it contributes heavily to the body's defenses against microorganisms by transporting enzymes, hormones, and antibodies throughout the body. Finally, the circulatory system removes waste products such as carbon dioxide and other metabolic waste. The circulatory system is made up of the heart, the blood vessels, and the blood.

Blood is much more than a mere liquid. It contains not only plasma, but also billions of cells. The fluid portion of the blood is called plasma. The amount of blood in the body depends on the amount of excess body fat: the less fat there is in the body, the more blood the body will have per pound of body weight. About 55 percent of total blood volume is made up of plasma; the rest consists of blood cells.

Blood Cells

The three types of blood cells:

- Red Blood Cells

- White Blood Cells

- Platelets

Red Blood Cells

Red blood cells are very small in size. Indeed, more than 3,000 of them could be placed side by side in a one-inch space. These tiny cells are manufactured in the bone marrow and possess no nucleus. Red blood cells transport oxygen from the lungs to the cells and remove carbon dioxide from the cells to the lungs. Red blood cells are made from hemoglobin. One hemoglobin atom is made up of globin and iron. Women possess less hemoglobin than men. Any person with less than 12 grams hemoglobin content is diagnosed as having anemia. A red blood cell's life expectancy is believed to be 120 days. As they become older, the membranes of red blood cells become fragile and eventually rupture, causing the cell to break apart within the capillaries. The iron content of the resultant red cell fragments is transported to the bone marrow, where it is used in the production of new red blood cells. Normally, over 100 million red blood cells are destroyed every hour, with a similar amount of new cells being manufactured to keep the number of red blood cells relatively constant at about 4 ½ to 5 ½ million cells per cubic meter of blood. To maintain the number of red blood cells in a healthy range, the blood must supply the bone marrow (where red blood cells are produced) with iron, amino acids, vitamin B12, and copper. In the case where the diet lacks vitamin B12 or the digestive system fails to absorb vitamin B12, an anemia (pernicious anemia) develops in the body.

White Blood cells

White blood cells, which are formed in the thymus gland, contribute to the body's defense mechanisms through their ability to carry out phagocytosis. During phagocytosis, white blood cells ingest and digest microorganisms and other foreign particles. Additionally, some white blood cells have the ability to move out of the capillaries by squeezing through the intercellular space of the capillary wall. They can then move towards microorganisms that have invaded the body's tissues. Some white blood cells are responsible for synthesizing and secreting circulatory antibodies as well.

Antibodies

From the thymus gland, in which they are formed, white blood cells enter the blood stream and then circulate to the lymphatic tissues where they take up residence. The white blood cells go on to multiply and form new lymphatic tissues.

Antibodies, which prevent infection, are produced by white blood cells residing in the lymphatic tissue.

White blood cells generally live between three and twelve days. Phagocytes and microorganisms destroy some white blood cells. In a healthy system, there are approximately 5,000 to 9,000 white blood cells per cubic millimeter. The white blood cell count changes in a state of disease as the number of white blood cells is increased when there is an infection in the body.

Platelets

Platelets look like small fragments of cells and are, like red blood cells, formed in the red bone marrow. They have a lifespan of seven to ten days. The major function of the platelets is to aid in the blood clotting mechanism.

Blood Types

The term "blood type" refers to the type of antigens present in the red blood cell membranes. An antigen is any substance, which is capable of forming antibodies when introduced into the body or into the bloodstream. Antigens A, B, and pH are the most important blood antigens as far as transfusion is concerned. Human blood belongs to one of four types and, in addition, is either RH positive or RH negative. Blood types are named according to the antigens present in the red cell's membranes.

They are:

Type A	Type AB
Type B	Type O

Plasma

Plasma is the liquid part of blood. It is a clear, straw-colored fluid that consists of 90% water and 10% solutes. The majority of these solutes are proteins while the remaining amount includes glucose, creatine, lactic acid, oxygen, carbon dioxide, hormones, and enzymes. The protein in plasma appears in the form of three main compounds: albumins, globulins, and fibrinogen. Plasma proteins are very important. Fibrinogen and albumin play key roles in the blood clotting mechanism, whereas globulins function as essential components of the immunity mechanism. All plasma proteins contribute to the maintenance of normal blood viscosity, volume, and osmotic pressure.

Blood Clotting

The purpose of blood clotting is to plug up the ruptured blood vessels so as to stop bleeding and prevent the loss of vital bodily fluid. Due to the obvious importance of this function, the mechanism for producing blood clotting must be swift and sure when needed. The blood clotting mechanism consists of a series of chemical reactions that take place in a definite and rapid sequence. In one or two seconds clumps of platelets adhere to any portion of a blood vessel and their membranes rupture, releasing enzymes, which trigger the blood clotting.

Three processes are involved in blood clotting:

- Prothrombin is converted to thrombin.

- Thrombin is converted to fibrinogen.

- Fibrinogen is converted to fibrin.

All plasma proteins are produced in the liver. In order for liver cells to synthesize the protein prothrombin at a normal rate, the blood must contain an adequate amount of Vitamin K. To complete the process of blood clotting there is a need for Vitamin K. Vitamin K is produced by certain bacteria in the colon.

The following factors may prevent blood clotting:

- The platelets do not adhere to the blood vessels. Consequently, they do not release the enzymes that trigger the blood clotting mechanism.

- The presence of Heparin, a natural constituent of the blood, acts as anti-thrombin or as an anti-clotting agent. Therefore, thrombin cannot be converted into fibrin to promote clotting.

The following factors hasten the blood clotting process:

- A rough spot develops on the lining of blood vessels, causing slow blood flow.

- The accumulation of blood cholesterol causes plaque development in the blood vessels.

- Immobility causes blood flow to slow down as movement decreases. This is the reason physicians insist that bed-ridden patients must either move or be moved frequently.

22

YOUR HEART

This chapter deals with the effect of exercise and physical activity on the heart, pulse rate, and blood pressure.

The Human Heart

The human heart is made up of four chambers. It is shaped and sized roughly like a man's closed fist. The heart lies to the left of the mid-line of the chest and has its own covering, a loose fitting sac called the pericardium. This sac is made of tough white fibrous tissue.

The pericardium consists of two parts: a fibrous portion and a serous portion. The fibrous portion, called the fibrous sac, is not attached to the heart itself, but fits loosely around the heart. The resultant space between the heart and the sac is called the "pericardial space" it contains five drops of lubricating fluid (pericardial fluid). The pericardial sac serves to protect the heart against friction.

Structure and function of the heart

The function of the heart is to pump blood in order to supply oxygen and nutrients to cells and tissues. The wall of the heart is made up of three layers of tissue. The bulk of the wall is comprised of specially constructed muscle tissue known as cardiac muscle. The interior of the heart is divided into two upper chambers and two lower chambers. The upper chambers (cavities) are termed atria and the lower chambers ventricles. Of these, the ventricles are larger and thicker-walled than the atria as they perform a heavier pumping function than the atria. For the same reason, the walls of the left ventricle are thicker than those of the right ventricle. The reason it is thicker is in order to produce more force to pump the blood into the arteries.

Heart Valves

The valves are like mechanical devices that permit the flow of blood in a single direction. There are four sets of valves and they are crucial for the normal functioning of the heart. Two of these four sets are the cusped valves, located in the heart, just at the openings between the atria and ventricles. The other two sets of valves, the bicuspid valves, are located inside the pulmonary artery and the great aorta, just as they arise from the right and left ventricles, respectively. The cuspid valves allow blood to flow from the atria into the ventricles, but prevent blood from flowing back up into the atria once in the ventricle. When the ventricles contract, blood is forced against the cuspid valves closing them, thereby, insuring the upward movement of blood. The cuspid valves prevent backflow of the blood. Any one of the four valves may lose the ability to close completely, resulting in a condition known as "vitral inefficiency." Vitral inefficiency permits blood to leak back into the chamber of the heart from which it came. When the bicuspid valve does not close completely it creates a backflow leak. The sound of the backflow leak is called "murmur."

Blood Supply

The heart receives blood by way of two small vessels, the right and left coronary arteries, which have two main branches. The coronary arteries supply both the heart's ventricles with blood. The left ventricle receives the most abundant blood supply of the two as it performs most of the work and, therefore, requires a greater quantity of oxygen and nutrients than the right ventricle.

Conduction System

Four structures comprise the conduction system of the heart:

- The Sino-atrial node (S.A. node)

- The Atrioventricular node (A.V. node)

- The Atrioventricular bundle

- The Purkinje Fibers

Each of the above structures plays an important role in the conduction of impulses and the rhythm of the heart. The S.A. node, or pacemaker, is made up of cells located in the right aerial wall near the opening of the superior vena cava.

In the absence of nerve stimulation, the S.A. node will contract indefinitely at a constant rate. As the cells of the S.A. node contract, they send impulses through to the myocardium, initiating a heartbeat. In this way, the S.A. node sets the basic pace of the heart rate and is referred to as "the pacemaker." It should be noted however, that the rate set by the S.A. node can be modified by the hormones and the nervous system. Impulses start in the S.A. node and speed through atrial muscle fibers in all directions, causing arterial contraction. When these impulses reach the atrioventricular node (A.V. node), they are relayed to the ventricles by way of the atrioventricular bundle and the Purkinje fibers. The impulses then cause the ventricles to contract.

Cardiac System

A complete contraction and relaxation sequence of both the atria and ventricles is called a "cardiac cycle." In a cardiac cycle, two atria contract simultaneously and then relax. Then both ventricles contract and relax, as well. The contracting force of the atria completes the emptying of blood from the atria into the ventricles. Then they relax as they are filled with blood. At this time (atria emptied of blood and ventricles filled with blood) the cuspid valve is open and the atria relax as blood enters them through the veins. The heart, clearly, neither contracts nor relaxes as an entire unit but does so in stages of a cycle; each stage performed by different chambers (atria and ventricles) at different times.

Heart Sounds

The heart makes certain sounds during each cycle that are described as resembling: "lubb-dubb" through a stethoscope. The incomplete closing of the bicuspid valve produces the well-known "lubb-dubb" sound. This sound is important because it reveals the condition of the valves: open or closed.

Blood Vessels

There are three types of blood vessels in the body:

- Arteries

- Veins

- Capillaries

Arteries

The artery is a vessel that carries blood away from the heart. All arteries carry oxygenated blood, with the exception of the pulmonary artery, which carries deoxygenated blood. The walls of the arteries are comprised of elastic fibers, which give them the ability to expand and relax, like a coil.

Veins

The vein is a vessel that transports blood *to* the heart. The pulmonary vein is an exception. It carries blood *away* from the heart to the lungs and contains deoxygenated blood

Capillaries

The capillaries are very small vessels that, because of their miniature size, are able to carry blood from arteries to veins. Since the main purpose of the blood is to transport essential materials to and from the cells, the capillaries are functionally very important. It is in the capillaries that the collection and deliveries of these materials takes place.

Blood Pressure

Blood pressure is the force by which blood is pushed out of the heart.
Blood pressure has two components:

• Systolic Blood Pressure

• Diastolic Blood Pressure

The systolic blood pressure refers to the force with which the blood pushes against the arterial walls when the ventricles contract. The diastolic blood pressure refers to the blood's force when the ventricles are relaxed. Systolic blood pressure gives valuable information about the force/strength/capacity of the left ventricle. Diastolic blood pressure provides valuable information about the resistance of the blood vessels. Clinically, diastolic blood pressure is considered more important than systolic blood pressure, because it indicates the degree of pressure or strain to which the walls of the blood vessels are constantly subjected. It also reflects the condition of the peripheral vessels since diastolic pressure rises and falls with peripheral resistance: if the arteries are hardened, for example, this indicates both increased peripheral resistance and higher diastolic blood pressure.

Blood in the arteries of an average adult exerts a pressure of 120 mm during the systolic phase of ventricular contraction and 80 mm during the diastolic phase. Systolic blood pressure measuring over 130 mm is considered to be a health risk and diastolic blood pressure over 90 mm is considered a high pressure. High diastolic blood pressure is very dangerous and may cause sudden death.

Pulse

Pulse is the result of the alternate expansion and recoiling of an artery, which is produced by the contraction and relaxation of the heart. Two factors are responsible for the existence of a pulse:

• The inflow or "injection" of blood from the heart into the aorta, resulting in alternating increases and decreases in the level of pressure in that vessel.

• The elasticity of the arterial walls, making it possible for them to expand and recoil with each injection of blood.

How to locate your pulse

The pulse can be felt wherever an artery lies over the bone, near the surface of the skin. Specific locations where the pulse can be easily felt include:

• Radial artery at the wrist

• Temporal artery in front of the ear

• Common carotid artery on either side of the neck

• Facial artery at the lower margin of the lower jawbone, in line with the corners of the mouth.

23

YOUR RESPIRATORY SYSTEM

Breathing supplies the body with oxygen. This chapter describes the structure, location and function of the lungs and how daily exercise benefits the respiratory system.

The Lungs

Both the left lung and right lung are cone-shaped organs located in the chest cavity. The left lung is divided into two lobes while the right lung consists of three lobes. Internally, each lung is composed of millions of microscopic alveoli with related ducts and bronchi. The exchange of gases between blood and air takes place in the lungs. The structure of the lungs makes this exchange possible because an open airway branches into millions of thin-walled alveoli, enveloped in networks of capillaries. As a result of this arrangement, it is possible for a large amount of oxygen to be quickly *loaded into* the blood and for large amounts of carbon dioxide to be quickly *unloaded from* the blood to the lungs and out.

Physiology of the lungs

Two types of respirations take place in the lungs:

- External Respiration

- Internal Respiration

Air moves in and out of the lungs for the same reason that blood flows in the vessels, because oxygen pressure outside the body is greater than oxygen pressure in the blood. That difference in gradient pressure makes the oxygen enter the blood. A gas pressure gradient, in the case of air movement, occurs when the atmospheric pressure is greater than the pressure within the lungs, and air flows in a direction of less pressure; i.e., down the gradient, from the atmosphere into the lungs. Inspiration occurs when pressure is greater than the atmospheric pressure and air again moves down the gas pressure gradient, but in the opposite direction, from the lungs into the atmosphere. The pressure gradients are established by changes in the size of the thoracic cavity, changes brought about by the contraction and relaxation of the respiratory muscles.

Other muscles may also contract at the same time elevating the sternum and ribs, thereby enlarging the thorax both from front to back and from side to side. The increase in the size of the thorax causes air to move inside the lungs. During expiration, the size of the thorax is decreased and pressure is put on the lungs as air moves out of the lungs and into the atmosphere. A device called the Spiro meter is used to measure the amount of air exchanged in breathing. The term "tidal air" refers to the amount of air normally exhaled after breathing. The normal volume of tidal air is 500 milliliters. After normal inspiration, you can force still more air out of the lungs. The largest amount of air that you can forcibly expire after normal inspiration is called expiratory reserve (volume= 1,000-1,200 milliliters). The average inspiratory reserve volume is about 3.3 liters, vital capacity. Vital capacity refers to the largest possible expiration after the largest possible inspiration. The size of vital capacity depends on several factors:

- Size of the thoracic cavity

- Size of the rib cage

- Posture

- Certain diseases viz. emphysema and lung cancer

Blood transports oxygen and carbon dioxide as solutes. Immediately upon entering the blood, both of these solutes dissolve in the plasma. Yet, since fluids (such as blood) can only hold small amounts of gases in solution, most of the oxygen and carbon dioxide rapidly forms a union with other blood chemicals. In this way, large volumes of gases can be transported. The amount of oxygen that can be transported to the cells depends on the amount of hemoglobin in the blood: blood that has less hemoglobin transports less oxygen.

Exchange of gases in the lungs

The exchange of gases takes place between the alveolar and venous blood, flowing through the lung capillaries. Gas moves in both directions through the alveolar capillary membrane. The oxygen enters the blood from the alveolar air because of the high pressure of oxygen and carbon dioxide.

Exchange of gases in the tissues

The exchange of gases takes place in the arterial blood flowing through the tissues, capillaries, and cells. It occurs because of the principle already noted, that gases move in and out of tissues based on the differences in the gas pressure.

Exercise and Respiration

A healthy respiratory system has two major characteristics:

- During normal breathing more air is exchanged between the atmosphere and the lungs.

- More aerovalas (air sacs) are opened creating more surface area in the lungs so that the exchange of gasses (oxygen and carbon dioxide) takes place much faster.

Sedentary living along with aging has a tremendous effect on the number of air sacs present. Their numbers go down as time goes on. The ability of a person to take more oxygen in and release carbon dioxide out depends on the number of opened air sacs available. In sedentary people more air sacs are closed and they cannot take in sufficient oxygen, leaving them feeling sluggish and tired. Daily exercise has a major benefit not only to the lungs but also to other organs of the body because all organs need oxygen to metabolize nutrients and to generate energy for their activities in the respiratory system and for general physical activities.

Daily Exercise:

- Increases the volume air, exchanged between atmosphere and lungs

- Helps to open up more air sacs and increases the exchange of oxygen and carbon dioxide. As a result of this more oxygen becomes available to the tissues.

- Strengthens the respiratory muscles

- Increases the depth of the breathing. More air per minute enters the lungs than in sedentary lungs. As a result of this physically active people breathe less per minute than inactive and less active people.

- Helps to prevent respiratory problems such as infection, allergies, asthma, and cancer of the lungs

24

YOUR MUSCULAR SYSTEM

Strength Development

The ability to adjust to changing conditions in the environment is crucial to our survival. Motion, not surprisingly, plays a major role in this adjustment. Although most of our bodies systems play some role in achieving movement, it is the muscular and skeletal systems particularly, acting in unison, that produce the most motion. Bones and joints naturally support the body's movements, but cannot successfully produce action without the aid of the muscles. The elasticity, contractibility and extendibility of muscles make motion possible.

Isotonic and Isometric Exercise

The two major categories of motion are:

- **Isotonic.**

  Locomotion, i.e., the movement of parts of the body and changes in the size of the length of the muscles such as walking and running

- **Isometric.**

  Contraction of the muscles is where the size of the muscle does not change, i.e., contraction and relaxation of the iris muscle of the eyes. This form of contraction and relaxation permits just the right amount of light to enter the eye, whereas the contraction and relaxation of the muscles of the digestive tract promotes essential bodily functions involving digestion and elimination. The contraction of the heart muscle keeps the blood circulating. These are all isometric activities because the length of the muscles is not changing.

Muscular strength plays a vital role in controlling our balance, protecting our joints and in maintaining joint flexibility. Lack of muscular strength can lead to chronic pain later in life especially back pain and may contribute to stress fractures. Ages ago, both men and women had more effective muscular systems because they walked more, carried and pushed more often, and performed a wider range of daily physical activities. Today, we drive everywhere and seldom carry anything heavier than a grocery bag from the car to the house. By not using our muscles, we lose much of their strength. By age forty, we can lose up to 40% of our muscular strength if we remain inactive or sedentary. In fact, the first signs of aging takes place in the muscular system long before we recognize the signs of our external aging. Therefore, it is very important that we engage in some form of physical activity that can maintain or improve our muscular strength. The best way to achieve this is through a program of weight training activities.

Four principles for an effective workout

There are four general principles that should be followed to ensure the greatest possible benefits result.

- **Principle One**

  Training programs should provide a progressive heavy overload on the specific muscle groups targeted for strengthening. A minimal overload will result in minimal strength, but a maximal overload produces maximal strength.

- **Principle Two**

  To develop actual strength, it is important to exercise with heavy weights and with less repetition. The loads must be progressively increased to keep pace with strength development.

- **Principle Three**

  Exercise larger muscle groups before smaller muscle groups.

- **Principle Four**

  Allow for adequate recovery time between each exercise. The methodology of overloading causes muscle fatigue. When muscles are tired it becomes difficult to advance in your training program. Therefore it is important to follow a routine that exercises different groups of muscles. For example, first do a leg exercise, then an arm exercise or if using universal equipment perform a leg press followed by a bench press. This method will increase muscular endurance and strength development and prevent early fatigue.

Muscular Definition

Human muscle accumulates fat between the skin and muscle as well as "inside" the muscle, unlike species such as chickens or birds. We can appear to have lost weight when we diet by losing the weight between the skin and muscle, but we do not gain definition until we lose the fat inside the muscles. In order to achieve muscle definition, you need a different method of weight training. First, you must reduce the weight load and increase the repetitions. Next, the repetitions must be in groups of 12 to 15 repetitions. Then do four sets of repetitions with a brief rest between each repetition. For example, if you want to create definition in your biceps do the following:

- Lower weight

- High repetition (15 reps)

- More sets (5 sets)

Muscle Structure

Muscles, like other tissues, are made up of cells. Because these cells are especially long and narrow, we refer to them as "fibers." Muscle fibers possess a structure unique unto themselves. The most common structural arrangement features small fibers, or myofibrils, packed closely together in a sac called the sarcoplasma. Muscle fibers not only contain carbohydrates, protein, fat, and water, but also, actin, myosin, troponin, and myoglobin. Myoglobin is a protein. Myoglobin is especially important because it is responsible for supplying the muscle fibers with oxygen from the blood.

The proper functioning of a muscle is based upon adequate circulation. Each local muscle that is involved in physical activity must receive an appropriate supply of oxygen as well as an appropriate removal of its waste products. Both the supply of oxygen and the removal of waste are accomplished via blood flow through the muscle. Consequently, the capillary network is essential to the development of muscular endurance. In addition, muscles contain myoglobin, a pigment that does not require significant pressure to combine with oxygen in the blood. Myoglobin, therefore, acts as an important storage place for oxygen in the muscles. Some muscles contain more myoglobin than others and, consequently, appear redder under histlgic examination. It is felt that such red, myoglobin-rich muscles are better equipped for high endurance; i.e., aerobic activity than paler muscles, whose functions seem better served for rapid-action; i.e., anaerobic activity. In light of the important physiological implications of muscular coloration, it is preferable to refer to "fast twitch" and "slow twitch" muscles instead "pale/white" and "red" muscles, respectively. Fast twitch (white colored) muscles are more capable of high-speed activity over a short duration of time, whereas slow twitch (red colored) muscles are, as a rule, better able to sustain long-term activity. The high myosin concentration and high glycolic activity in the fast twitch muscles lies at the root of the physiological differences between the muscle types. Very little can be done to change fast twitch muscles into slow twitch or *vice versa*. Individuals are born with either more fast twitch or more slow twitch muscles: these characteristics are based on genetics and not training.

Energy sources for muscular activity

Contrary to the belief that fuel for exercise is composed primarily of carbohydrates, energy for physical work comes from the breakdown of both fats and carbohydrates. It is becoming increasingly evident that fat metabolism is an important energy source, and that the fat used comes from free fatty acids hydrolyzed from the triglycerides of the adipose tissue by the enzyme lipase. Fatty acids diffuse into the blood and are transported to the muscles where the fatty acids yield energy after undergoing the process of oxidation. Since forty percent of the calories in the average diet come from fats and about the same amount come from carbohydrates, it has been estimated that between thirty and fifty percent of ingested carbohydrates are converted to triglycerides. These statistics signify that anywhere from two-thirds to three-fourths of all energy provided by the diet, actually comes from fats rather than carbohydrates. Carbohydrates are used for short, fast, strenuous bouts of activity. Fats, in contrast, are used for light and moderate bouts of prolonged activity. Furthermore, the efficiency of conversion for fats is different than for carbohydrates. Fats require 2.01 liters of oxygen for their oxidation in contrast to carbohydrates, which need only 0.75 liters of oxygen. Fat, however, produces twice as much energy per gram as carbohydrates and may be stored in large quantities in the adipose tissues. It should be added, nonetheless, that fat cannot be converted to carbohydrates. By increasing your consumption of complex carbohydrates you can influence the efficiency of your ability to exercise (i.e. increased speed, strength, endurance). However, repeated exertion reduces a muscle's ability to contract, and fatigue results. The fatigue process stems from three potential areas:

• The synapses of the central nervous system

- The nerve impulses

- The muscle itself

Muscular Training

Regarding muscular training, individuals are engaged in one of two types of exercise:

- **Isotonic exercise**—this form of exercise is involved in raising and lowering a load.

- **Isometric exercise**—this form of exercise requires that a static contraction be held against resistance over time.

Isotonic exercise is a progressive resistance exercise, usually given in either sets or a number of repetitions (ranging from 6-10). Since strict standards have not been established, a great deal of individual preference exists. Six repetitions done over three sets, performed three times per week are suggested as the optimal training combination.

Isometric exercise, because it does not improve circulation and may lead to increased blood pressure, has not proven to be as effective as isotonic exercise.

Strength vs. Endurance

It is very important to appreciate the distinction between strength and endurance. A test of muscular strength, for example, might involve concentrating one's maximum effort on lifting a single heavy weight, whereas a test of muscular endurance might involve performing a large number of push ups or chin-ups. Both muscular strength and muscular endurance are important in their own ways and each possesses different corresponding physiological requirements. Muscular endurance must be supported by circulation and energy needs will be different than those required for a test of single-effort muscular strength. It is typical to develop strength by de-emphasizing endurance, such as by using a weight-training program that involves high resistance but few repetitions.

Endurance development involves low resistance and high repetition. This technique is very important for two reasons:

- It improves the circulation to the muscles

- It increases the capillarization of the muscles

Low repetition coupled with a high resistance does not effectively promote circulation in the muscles nor does it increase capillarization. In contrast, low repetition and high resistance causes hypertrophy of the muscles. Hypertrophy results in increased strength and muscle mass; it is attributed to the long-term effects of heavy resistance exercise. New muscle fibers do not form as a result of hypertrophy, but the myofibrillar portion of the muscle is increased, enhancing the contractibility of the muscle fibers. Increased contractibility leads to improved muscular strength.

Strength training can be achieved through the use of progressive resistance exercise. The aim is to increase the size of the individual muscle fibers, specifically by increasing the nitrogen components of the myofilament. A strength-training regiment also increases the density of the myofilaments within the muscle cells, making the development of tension greater after a training session. The same changes occurring in the muscle cells take place in the connective tissues, ligaments, and tendons as well.

25

YOUR BODY TEMPERATURE DURING EXERCISE

Exercise and heat exchange

Sweating is a defense mechanism designed to protect the body from overheating in a hot environment or during strenuous exercise. The sweating mechanism is carried out through the sweat glands, of which there are two types:

- Eccrine

- Apocrine

Eccrine sweat glands are found all over the body, but primarily in the palms of the hands, the soles of the feet, and in the head. The eccrine glands secrete chloride, urine, and lactic acid. The salt concentration of eccrine secretions ranges from 0.1 to 0.37 g. The eccrine gland's function is to control body temperature.

Apocrine glands are located around hair follicles and are primarily found in the auxiliary and pubic regions. The strange odor known to emanate from these regions is characteristic of apocrine sweat. The apocrine glands are stimulated by emotional stress.

Physical exercise increases body temperature and causes sweating. One of the essential requirements for the sweating mechanism is that sufficient water be present in the body, which, in turn, means there must be a comparable intake of water in order to compensate for the losses that occur during sweating. Rehydrate your body by drinking fluids. Failure to keep pace with the loss of water can result in dehydration. Under conditions of dehydration your ability to sweat is restricted, leading to impaired temperature regulation and very high body temperature. Under these conditions heat stroke may ensue, making it necessary to provide water to athletes performing for long durations or at high temperatures.

We are approximately 65 per cent to 70 per cent water. A loss of only 2 per cent of water can reduce physical and mental performance by up to 20 per cent. Dehydration causes the chemical processes in the body that require water to shut down, destabilizing the function of the internal organs. For example, a marked reduction in potassium, which regulates the heart can cause stroke. Only oxygen is more important than water for survival.

Exercise and Metabolism

All muscular activities require energy. Energy is derived from the oxidation of foods in the body. In the body, foods are stored either as fat or as glycogen. Since there is no stored oxygen in the body, measuring the oxygen consumption constitutes the most convenient way to determine the energy cost of physical exercise. Physical activities may be classified according to the amount of energy required to perform them. It has been shown that the minute-by-minute energy utilization is accurately reflected in oxygen intake, at least until high levels of work are reached. When the muscle calls on metabolic mechanisms, which release energy temporarily without utilizing oxygen, this results in excess oxygen consumption during recovery and is known as oxygen debt. The total energy cost of high levels of physical exercise is properly calculated as the sum of the oxygen consumption during physical work plus the sum of oxygen consumption occurring after work. High levels of activity that can be maintained over long periods of time are generally referred to as aerobic work. Under the conditions of aerobic work, the heart and lungs keep up with the oxygen requirements, but when the intensity of exercise rises and the heart and lungs are no longer able to supply enough oxygen to meet the demands of exercise, oxygen debt occurs. Such activities can only be maintained for a relatively short period of time, usually less than five minutes, and are referred to as anaerobic activities, such as the hundred-yard dash.

In an exercise such as walking, the person's weight and walking speed play an important role in energy consumption, whereas age and genetic factors such as race and sex have limited effect. Furthermore, training has no effect on the energy expenditure of walking as nearly all active adults have already developed a high level of skill in this activity. In exercises such as running or swimming, however, it is easy to show that the building of skill through repetition, especially performed by people who have had more experience running or swimming, reduces their energy expenditure, enabling them to run or swim a given distance at a higher speed. The practice and attention given by athletes to form and skill will improve their performance. It has been shown that physical activity can be most efficiently performed in an aerobic state; i.e., slow speed of muscular contraction.

Physical activities requiring a high speed of muscular contraction only waste energy. If a muscle is contracted and then stretched, the muscle will absorb energy. Such exercise can be sustained for a longer period of time, with very little energy expenditure and with a small amount of lactic acid accumulation and fatigue. During maximal work, oxygen consumption stabilizes and no longer increases with a rise in the intensity of the workload. It is believed that at maximal work, the cardiovascular and respiratory systems are unable to increase their oxygen deliveries to the working muscles. The additional energy needed to carry on this kind of work must come from the metabolism of carbohydrates. Exercising above maximum capacity will require more oxygen than your cardiovascular system can supply and causes "oxygen debt." Athletes like long distance runners who are able to perform tasks requiring high-energy expenditure over a prolonged period must have maximum oxygen intake. Short distance runners, in contrast, benefit from the capacity to accumulate a large oxygen debt. It has been shown that obtaining energy through the oxygen debt mechanism is an insufficient process because it increases the cost of work. The oxygen cost of running at a steady pace over a specified distance or of starting that distance fast and ending at a slower pace, indicates that both strategies are, in fact, wasteful of the runner's energy. The given distance can be covered in a shorter time if the runner starts slowly and finishes the race with a sprint. Such a plan will be more effective for a long-distance race.

All muscular activities are carried out using energy supplied by food. The energy used by muscles, however, appears to be drawn from high-energy bonds, built up by a complex chain of chemical reactions originating with the actual oxidation of food energy itself. It is this energy that is stored in the muscles.

Energy sources for endurance training

The two main sources are:

- Glycogen

- Fats (high-energy bonds)

Glycogen, which is basically glucose, provides energy for short distance running and high-speed activities. High-energy bonds provide energy for longer and slower pace activities such as jogging and fast walking.

26

CLASSIFICATION OF EXERCISE

This chapter will provide you with an understanding of how the circulatory, respiratory, and muscular systems work in conjunction during exercise. I discuss a variety of conditioning exercises and the effect of proper nutrition on athletic performance, including weight lifting and marathon running.

Ranges of Intensity

Physical activities can be classified into three groups based on their oxygen requirements:

- **Moderate** physical activity, which requires oxygen at a rate of three times the resting oxygen requirement for the basal metabolic rate. Such activities raise the pulse rate to 140 beats per minute. Examples include fast walking and jogging.

- **Hard** physical activity, which requires three to eight times the basal metabolic rate and raises the pulse rate to above 140 beats per minute. Examples include running and skiing.

- **Maximal** physical activity, which requires the maximum performance of both the cardiovascular and respiratory systems and raises the pulse rate above 160 beats per minute, leading to oxygen debt. Examples include competitive level skiing and cycling.
Note: Class One and Two (Moderate and Hard) physical activities encompass the great majority of physical activities.

Factors affecting oxygen intake

When a person performs a physical exercise and maintains it for a long period of time, the following oxygen consumption will apply:

Oxygen consumption will go up if the activity is continued for about three to five minutes. It is followed by a constant rate of oxygen consumption. This latter phase is referred to as the steady state with regard to oxygen consumption. After exercise has stopped, the rate of oxygen intake continues at a rate above the basal rate for a period of time depending on the intensity of the exercise being performed. The total oxygen consumption in excess of the basal requirement after exercise is referred to as oxygen debt. The size of one's oxygen debt after exercise is directly related to the lag in oxygen intake at the beginning of exercise to reach steady state; the oxygen intake must be equal to the oxygen requirement in order to continue exercise for extended periods of time.

Metabolism during exercise

The metabolic activities of the body during physical exercise differ greatly from the body's metabolic activities during rest. The metabolism that occurs during exercise involves interplay among three factors:

• The supply of oxygen to the muscles

• The supply of fuel to the muscles: glucose and fatty acids

• The ability of the lungs to pass oxygen on to the blood flowing to the muscles

The glucose used as muscle fuel is drawn mainly from glycogen stored within the muscle itself. Fatty acids come, in part, from fat located inside the muscles and, in part, from adipose tissues.

Of the three factors mentioned above, oxygen supply is the limiting factor. In order to use an unlimited supply of body fat for fuel, the lungs must supply ample amounts of oxygen to break down fatty acids. This is an aerobic process. When muscular activity is so intense that the energy demand of the muscles becomes more than their available oxygen supply, it is no longer possible to rely solely on the aerobic process of fat metabolism to provide the needed energy. The muscles must draw more heavily on their own limited supply of glucose. Glucose can be metabolized without oxygen to produce energy for muscular activity. When the body produces energy from glucose in the absence of oxygen, a waste product called lactic acid appears in the muscle. Accumulation of lactic acid in the muscles causes fatigue and pain; lactic acids can only be disposed of when oxygen becomes available to the muscles again.

Regarding their use of energy fuels, muscles are classified in two groups:

- Muscles specializing in anaerobic activity

- Muscles specializing in aerobic activity

The muscles specializing in anaerobic processes are involved in intense activities such as the exertion that occurs in weightlifting. A weightlifter's muscles must tighten and remain tight for many seconds at a time. Muscles specializing in such efforts are known as "fast-twitch" muscle fibers. These fibers appear white under the microscope. They use glucose for energy. The second group of muscles is known as "slow-twitch" muscle fibers; they mainly burn fat as fuel and appear red when viewed under the microscope. Slow-twitch muscles contract and relax many times in the space of a few seconds and are used in such activities as playing basketball or long-distance running.

Energy and Nutrition

There is a strong correlation between nutrition and athletic performance. Regular exercise and optimal nutrition are both essential if one is to maintain a high quality of life. Glycogen and fat constitute the two main sources of fuel found in the body. Muscles also use fat circulated in the blood stream during exercise. During low or moderate intensity activities, muscle cells mainly use fat as fuel. During intense activity they use glycogen, and after glycogen is used up they use fat and small amounts of protein. The details are best illustrated by observing what goes on inside a marathon runner throughout the course of a race.

If the runner starts off without a warm-up, his or her muscles will begin using glycogen intensively as the individual's heart and lungs haven't started working hard enough to supply a sufficient amount of oxygen to support aerobic activity. Pyruvic, lactic, and other acids then begin to accumulate and within five minutes, 20 percent of the muscle's glycogen will have been burned up. However, the cardiovascular system will now have begun to work efficiently as aerobic activity starts to take over. The runner experiences this shift as a relief from his initial discomfort; a feeling commonly known as the "second wind." During this time the accumulated acids are oxidized, together with fat from both inside the muscle cells and from fatty acids released from adipose cells (excess fat deposits) elsewhere in the body. For as long as possible, the body burns a mixture of four fuels:

fat from the two sources already mentioned (intra-muscular and extra-muscular) and glucose from both inside and outside the muscle as well. Throughout the race, the muscles continue to require some glucose to support their activity.

A runner in prime condition is capable of using fat for the longest period of time even while exercising at a high level of intensity. As the level of intensity rises, however, the runner relies less on fat and increasingly on glycogen to supply his energy needs. After 40 to 60 minutes of racing, free fatty acids in the blood are at six times the levels at which they started, and, if the runner stops at any point after this, ketosis ensues.

A marathon race goes on for 26 miles but, after about 20 miles, the runner "hits the wall," experiencing a sudden and disabling fatigue. The only recourse available is to slow down, for from this point on, the intensity of the exercise can only be as great as the aerobic fuel (fat) can support. Glucose released from the liver may still supply some energy for muscular work; at this point the breakdown of protein tissue may also help maintain blood glucose, but it cannot keep up with the needs of a marathon runner at full tilt.

Marathon runners have learned the ultimate limit to their endurance lies in the amount of glycogen they can pack away in their muscles before a race. This knowledge has led to the practice of "glycogen loading," a technique that involves a specific pattern of diet and exercise designed to trick the muscles into storing more glycogen than they normally would. The extra glycogen stored in the muscles postpones the onset of exhaustion and prolongs the time during which the marathoner can run his fastest speed.

27

EXERCISE AND OXYGEN CONUMPTION

Energy requirements of exercise

During physical activity oxygen and nutrients must be supplied to the muscles by the blood in proportion to demand, while carbon dioxide and heat generated by increased rates of metabolism must be removed from the muscles. In order to accomplish this task, cardiac output and blood flow are redistributed so an adequate amount of blood can reach the working muscle and skin. Under sub-maximal exercise, oxygen consumption and cardiac output can be maintained at a steady state for long periods. During maximum exertion, however, oxygen consumption reaches a very high level and the blood can no longer provide a high level of oxygen to the working muscles. Under such conditions, exercise cannot be maintained for a long time. The maximum capacity of an individual depends on the maximum oxygen delivery to the heart and the working muscles, as well as the removal of carbon dioxide and heat from the muscles. Such factors as age, sex, and fitness can also influence the cardiovascular system's reaction to exercise.

Muscular activity increases blood circulation to the exercising muscles. This is an essential phenomenon because, if circulation to the muscles does not increase, muscular contractions cannot be sustained for any significant amount of time and as a result, exercise must stop. Increased circulation is needed for several reasons: First of which is to supply more oxygen to the muscles; secondly, to remove waste products *viz.* carbon dioxide and lactic acid, which would otherwise accumulate rapidly and impair the functioning of the muscle; and, thirdly, to create a greater dissipation of the heat generated by muscular activity.

During physical activity, a series of events takes place in the cardiovascular system. Firstly, muscular contraction involves the use of fuel stores, which are generally oxidized as energy. Because the body's stores of oxygen are minimal, the blood must continuously supply this fuel if the necessary oxidative processes are to proceed. Normally the energy of muscular contraction comes from the oxidation of glycogen into carbon dioxide and water; oxygen is not indispensable for contraction itself, but it is absolutely necessary for the recovery phase. When the oxygen supplied to the muscles during exercise becomes inadequate, lactic acid forms and overflows into the blood stream. Under such conditions, a metabolic steady state cannot be established or maintained. Exercise must be stopped otherwise fatigue sets in or the person loses consciousness.

Cardiovascular Adaptation

Three main changes take place in the cardiovascular system during exercise. They include changes in:

- **Cardiac Output.** The most important change in the functioning of the cardiovascular system during exercise is the increase in cardiac output: the total volume of blood expelled by the heart per minute. The greater output is brought about by an increase in both the number of heartbeats per minute and the volume of blood pumped with each heartbeat.

- **Heart Rate.** At rest, the heart rate is quite variable depending not only upon posture but also upon such factors as the emotional state of the individual. During an athletic contest, the heart rate rises before exercise begins; the faster heart rate may be associated with a proportional increase in cardiac output. In fact, it really depends on the athlete's anticipation of the coming exercise and suggests that cardiovascular responses during exercise are partly mediated by the central nervous system. The liberation of such hormones as epinephrine and especially norepinephrine, plays a role in the rise of the pulse rate. A heart rate, measuring over 200 beats per minute has been observed in subjects driving themselves to very high levels of performance, but under the normal conditions of hard exercise, the heart rate increases to about two and one half times the resting level. When exercise stops, the heart rate remains very close to the maximum attained at the end of exercise for a few seconds; then recovery sets in and the pulse rate gradually decreases. The state of recovery of pulse rate is associated with the level of conditioning of the athlete. Well-trained athletes have a faster recovery pulse rate than the untrained person.

- **Blood Pressure.** During exercise systolic blood pressure increases in direct proportion to the workload, whereas diastolic blood pressure does not change significantly. The return of blood pressure to the resting level during recovery is dependent upon the intensity of the exercise. After moderate short-duration exercise, systolic blood pressure drops rapidly to pre-exercise levels and remains constant thereafter; diastolic blood pressure, in contrast, does not change. Upon the completion of high intensity exercise, systolic blood pressure decreases rapidly to below the resting level (pre-exercise level). After thirty to forty minutes, the systolic blood pressure returns to its resting level.

Cardiac Output

One of the most important benefits of regular exercise is an increase in cardiac output and stroke volume. Cardiac output refers to the amount of blood ejected by the heart per minute. Stroke volume is the amount of blood ejected from the heart in a single heartbeat.

The increase in stroke volume is achieved by the following conditions:

- Strength and efficiency of the heart muscle

- Increase in the velocity of the blood flow produced by the heart in its capacity as a pump

- Increased diffusion of oxygen from the gaseous phase into the liquid phase in the blood stream.

- Increased diffusion of carbon dioxide from the blood into a gaseous phase in the lungs

- Diffusion of oxygen from the blood into the muscles

Effect of exercise on blood pressure

The long-term effects of regular exercise on high blood pressure in both men and women have been studied extensively. All studies have shown a significant reduction of systolic and diastolic blood pressures.

- These reductions are brought about in the following ways:

- A reduction of the blood cholesterol and an improvement in the elasticity of the arterial walls

- A reduced viscosity of the blood, which lowers the resistance of the blood flow

- A reduction of water retention, a factor responsible for high blood pressure

- Reduced levels of stress and tension, factors responsible for high blood pressure

Regular physical exercise results in a slowed pulse rate, lower blood cholesterol, a high capacity for work, and a faster rate of recovery.

Distribution of blood flow

During exercise the blood flow to the active muscles increases, while blood flow to the digestive system, the liver, and the kidneys decreases. Circulation to the brain, however, remains constant. The amount of blood available to the exercising muscles is limited by the blood flowing to the skin to permit cooling. Available blood is also limited by the blood supply to the respiratory muscles; i.e., the diaphragm and the muscles of the trunk.

Heat Dissipation

The adjustment of the cardiovascular system is very important to the process of removing the heat produced by physical activity. Since physical activity increases the production of heat by the muscles heat must be dissipated in order to maintain body temperature within a safe limit. The dissipation of heat during physical activity obviously becomes more important under conditions of heavy exercise or warm weather. Under such conditions, cutaneous vasodilation occurs and blood flow to the skin increases. The increase in the flow of blood to the skin is necessary, not only to ensure heat loss by conduction from the blood, but also to provide for the metabolic and water needs of the sweat glands. As sweating increases, a significant amount of water may be lost, resulting in dehydration. This places additional stress on the cardiovascular system because dehydration triggers a decrease in the circulating blood volume as well as a rise in the viscosity of the blood. When an individual exercises in a hot environment, especially under conditions of high humidity, sweating and heat conduction may not be sufficient to dissipate the heat produced by exercise. As a result the body temperature rises and cardiovascular responses such as heat and cardiac output continue to increase, but oxygen consumption remains constant. The ability to reach a high level of oxygen intake and to maintain a satisfactory body temperature constitutes two most important factors necessary to achieving superior athletic performance.

Cardiac output = **heart beat** x stroke **volume**

Effect of exercise on heart rate

Heart rate is dependant upon one's body posture and the psychological state. Under conditions of stress the pulse rate rises, whereas it falls during periods of relaxation. Regarding posture, the pulse rate is lower when one is in a lying position as opposed to standing. Temperature has an effect on pulse rate as well; a rise in temperature will result in a higher pulse rate.

During exercise, systolic blood pressure increases while diastolic blood pressure remains unchanged. When a steady rate of oxygen consumption is achieved, systolic blood pressure remains at a constant level. The steady rate of oxygen consumption and systolic blood pressure can be noticed in the presence of a continuously rising heart rate, which indicates an increased cardiac output. Systolic blood pressure returns to the resting level during the recovery phase of exercise. After moderate exercise of comparatively short duration, systolic blood pressure drops rapidly to pre-exercise levels and remains constant thereafter, but after hard exercise, systolic blood pressure decreases rapidly to below resting levels. The diastolic blood pressure remains unchanged. After 20-30 minutes of exercise, the systolic blood pressure returns to the resting level, depending, however, upon the intensity of the exercise.

28

NUTRITIONAL DEFICIENCY DISEASES

It is a common belief that aging is responsible for the majority of chronic illness that is prevalent in adulthood. However, that idea is false. Environmental factors pose greater health risks that few people recognize. For example, the water we drink, the air we breathe, chemical additives in our foods, and germs over time are damaging to our health. The problem we face is learning to control the environmental factors within our reach in order to balance the physiological effects of aging. Chronological aging itself is a normal and natural process. There are many people all over the world and here at home in the United States, ninety years of age and older, who remain healthy and active despite their advanced age. Then there are young people who have serious health conditions. Aging, for example does not cause diabetes. With exception to juvenile diabetes, Type II diabetes is mainly caused by the consumption of carbohydrate-rich foods and a high-sugar diet. Excessive consumption of carbohydrate-rich foods, especially cake, pie, ice cream, and pasta puts a tremendous burden on the pancreas to maintain a steady production of insulin in order to metabolize all the sugar you are putting into your system. If you continue these dietary habits, eventually these foods will exhaust the pancreatic gland resulting in the inability to produce enough insulin for the bodies needs and you become diabetic. The same goes for most other chronic diseases. Another example, high blood pressure is caused by obesity and high salt intake. Heart diseases are directly attributed to a high-fat diet and lack of exercise. Digestive disorders are linked to lack of fiber in the diet, stress, high-fat foods, and insufficient consumption of fruits and vegetables. Consequently, the old saying "we are what we eat" is true. If you want to live a longer and healthier life, you must recognize the value in controlling your environment and what you put into your mouth. You are only as old as your lifestyle makes you.

The questions then arise, "what is aging?" and "why do we age?" Aging is a slow decline of the human body as a normal sequence of life. If we adjust ourselves to this natural process we can virtually live disease-free. For example, insulin production declines as we age. Therefore it is important to monitor our carbohydrate intake so that we do not become diabetic. We lose muscle tissue as part of the aging process. By exercising and consuming more fish and low-fat foods we reduce our risk of developing heart disease. Digestive enzymes decline with age. Therefore, increase the fruits and vegetables and decrease the protein sources (meats) in the diet because fewer enzymes are needed to digest these foods. And, reduce salt to prevent elevated blood pressure. Our anti-aging and healthy longevity concepts are a matter of what we choose to believe. How you choose to manage your environment now will have lasting effects later in life.

Diabetes

Type II diabetes is caused by consuming high carbohydrate foods, including pasta, cake, rice, potato, and cookies. To be metabolized efficiently, these foods place a high demand on the pancreas to produce insulin. Continues consumption of these foods typically leads to diabetes. Diabetes is one of the major diseases in the United States. More than 500,000 new cases are diagnosed each year. The yearly medical cost of this disease is more than 20 billion dollars. Diabetes is a disorder in which not enough insulin is produced within the body to move the glucose into the cells and use it for energy. As a result of insufficient insulin, the blood sugar rises. There are two major types of diabetes:

• Insulin Dependent

• Non-insulin Dependent

Insulin Dependent—in insulin dependent diabetes, the pancreas does not make insulin. Without insulin, the body cannot utilize the sugar and must try to use fat for energy. Combustion of fat results in an acid waste called Ketosis. As ketones build up in the blood supply, a serious metabolic condition known as Ketoacidosis occurs. If this condition is not treated, it may result in death. This type of diabetes usually occurs in young children and is called Juvenile Onset Diabetes. Only 10 percent of all incidences of diabetes belong to this group.

Non-Insulin Dependent—in non-insulin dependent diabetes, the pancreas makes some insulin, but it is an insufficient amount. Those having this type of diabetes still require some insulin from outside sources for normalizing the blood sugar. Of all the cases of diabetes, 85 percent are non-insulin dependent. Most of the non-insulin dependent cases occur after age 20 as a result of overeating, lack of exercise and gaining weight. An excessive amount of body fat reduces the efficiency of insulin in the body.

Symptoms of Diabetes

- Frequent urination

- Extreme hunger

- Thirst

- Blurred vision

- Easy tiring

- Drowsiness

Treatment

A high fiber diet—consumption of more fresh vegetables, fruits, legumes (beans, peas, lentils) and complex carbohydrates are excellent sources of fiber. The fiber found in these foods reduces insulin requirements and lowers fasting blood sugar and triglycerides.

Reduction of high fat foods—these include the following items: bacon, salad dressing, fried foods, cold cuts, alcohol, gravy, nuts, salt and non-complex carbohydrates (cakes, cookies, pastry, and sugar products).

Hypoglycemia

Hypoglycemia is a low blood sugar that is related to excessive production of insulin.

Treatment—do not consume the following foods

Pastries	Coffee
Soft Drinks	Sugar Products

Eat six small meals per day. Meals must include carbohydrates and proteins.

Asthma

It is the inflammation of the windpipe that can be caused by MSG, shellfish, and additives in foods.

Treatment—avoid cheese, wine, vinegar, oranges, shrimp, gelatin, and, MSG.

Gout

It is caused by high uric acid in the blood primarily through a high intake of beans, shellfish and red meat.

Treatment—avoid foods from the following categories

- Beans, peas, spinach, mushrooms, lentils, and asparagus

- Pork, shellfish, and red meat

Consume more foods from the following categories

- Carbohydrate-rich foods such as rice, bread, potatoes and pasta

- Eggs, cheese, and fruits

- Drink more water

Constipation

Constipation is a problem of evacuation of the bowel, which is caused by slow movement of the feces through the large intestine. During a prolonged stay in the colon, the feces become dry and hard as the water content of the feces is increasingly absorbed. The food we eat plays a very important role in the movement of fecal materials. Foods high in fiber such as fruits, vegetables, whole wheat breads, rice, and potatoes absorb water along the intestinal tract, thereby producing bulk and stimulating defecation. It is important that a person should have a daily bowel movement so that the digestive system stays clean and prevents the growth of bacteria.

Causes of Constipation

Lack of exercise—is an important factor in constipation. Exercise stimulates the intestinal muscles and strengthens them so that when the wall of the digestive tract contracts, it produces a strong force and forces the residue down facilitating the process of defecation.

Insufficient water intake—water is absorbed by food residue and produces soft and bulky feces. Such residue can be moved easier down the tract. Therefore it is important that each person drinks at least four glasses of water per day.

Emotional stress—causes constriction of the blood vessels and spasms of the muscles around the large intestine. As a result the peristalsis movement slows down and the feces becomes dry and hard. This contributes to constipation.

Treatment—requires a four-fold approach.

- Increasing water intake to 3 to 4 glasses of water per day

- Participation in daily exercise—an exercise program should be 20 to 30 minutes of jogging or walking at least 5 times per week

- Consuming more fruits, vegetables, rice, legumes, and whole wheat bread

- Reducing stress—most effective methods are becoming involved in meditation or some form of a hobby.

Acne

Additives in food are the major cause acne.

Treatment—is a three-fold approach

- Wash face with warm water 5 times per day

- Take Vitamins A (20,000 I.U.), Vitamin C (1000 mg) and B Complex

- Eat more fresh fruits

Avoid—foundation-like cosmetics and foods or beverages sold in cans, bottles, and jars

Spastic Colon

Spastic colon is a common disorder of an unknown cause that does not appear to be any organic abnormality. It is the result of over stimulation of the intestinal nerve endings that cause irregular contraction of the bowel. There is a loss of rectal sensitivity that can cause either rapid transit through the bowel or constipation. It is usually accompanied by nausea, constipation, or diarrhea, which may alternate. Because of the spasms, the mass moves more irregularly along the intestinal tract.

Causes—of spastic colon are related to

- Emotional upset or a prolonged period of stress

- Excessive use of laxatives

- Excessive use of coffee or tea

- Excessive use of tobacco

- Excessive use of alcohol

- Frequent use of antibiotics

- Lack of regular sleep or rest

Symptoms—include heartburn, feeling full, flatulence, severe cramping and pain

Prevention—is a two-fold approach

- A high fiber diet is recommended. Fiber adds bulk to the stool; relieves constipation, and the pressure within the colon walls

- A low fat diet is recommended. Consumption of fat, especially saturated fat, causes bloatedness, gas, and at times, diarrhea

Poor Circulation

Poor circulation is caused by lack of exercise, weight gain, and a high fat diet.

Treatment—consists of exercising, reducing the fat content of your diet, losing weight and taking Vitamin E (800 IU) and Folic Acid (400 mcg)

Diarrhea

Diarrhea is the occurrence of frequent liquid stools. It is a symptom, not a disease. The passage of food through the intestinal tract is abnormally rapid. The residue passes through the colon so quickly that there is no chance for the fluid to be absorbed.

There are two types of diarrhea

• Functional

• Organic

Functional diarrhea—is less severe and may occur in any normal, healthy person.

Causes—some major causes of functional diarrhea are overeating, eating the wrong foods, fermentation caused by incomplete digestion, nervous tension, and drinking too much coffee

Organic Diarrhea—is usually caused by external poison, such as food poisoning or parasites. Sometimes it is attributed to an enzyme deficiency that results in impaired digestion and absorption.

Treatment—in both cases of diarrhea, nutritional treatment is the same.

• Provide a diet that leaves little residue

• In severe cases lasting 12 to 24 hours, fasting is essential to provide rest to the digestive tract.

• Replacement of the fluid and electrolytes

After 12 hours, simple foods such as dry toast and tea are given. Scraped raw apple or applesauce may be given every 4 hours. Vitamin B, Vitamin C, and fruit juice should be given. When diarrhea stops, regular food should be taken gradually.

Diet and Tumors

The link between diet and tumors is very strong. Tumors do not appear out of nowhere. It takes years to produce a tumor. First, the process starts when something alters the genetic makeup of cells. Chemicals, viruses and radiation can damage cells, but the most important damaging agent of all is oxygen. In all activities we do, we generate reactive oxygen molecules called free radicals. These free radicals bounce around cells and steal electrons from molecules and consequently damage the DNA of the cells.

In the beginning of life, plants were anaerobic. They lived in a world free of oxygen. As they evolved, they began turning carbon dioxide into oxygen. By doing so, they polluted their environment with free oxygen that threatened their existence. In order to survive, they were forced to develop defenses against free oxygen. Plants began to produce a variety of colors: red, green, yellow, orange, purple, and white. These colors were called phytochemicals, which gave plants their vivid hues.

Phytochemicals are key parts of the antioxidant defense system. In addition to resisting oxidation, they guard against viral attack and harsh climate. The variety of colors that you find in fruits and vegetables are the colors that plants have produced to fight against free radicals, which are known to cause tumors. Since the consumption of fruits and vegetables has declined during the past 50 years, the cancer rate has climbed significantly. The American Cancer Institute concluded that poor eating habits are responsible for the high rate of cancer in the United States.

In order to combat cancer, we must do the following

- Increase the consumption of a variety of fruits, such as oranges, bananas, pears, apples, and all fruits having rich colors

- Increase the consumption of vegetables, such as kale, spinach, cabbage, tomatoes, eggplant, cucumber, squash, onion, peppers, and other color varieties

Each of these vegetables and fruits provide a strong shield against tumors. It is very important that we include a variety of fruits and vegetables in our daily diet.

Breast Cancer

Excessive body fat works as an estrogen factory. Women are at a greater risk of developing breast cancer if their excess fat is deposited on the upper torso or in the abdominal area. Obesity is associated with higher mortality rates in women undergoing various forms of treatment for cancer. The less fat women have, the less estrogen their bodies will produce. Estrogen destroys the DNA of the cells and contributes to formation of cancerous cells. Dietary factors that reduce the risk of developing breast cancer include reducing red meat, high fat and starchy foods and increase consumption of fruits, vegetables and seafoods. Fruits and vegetables are very high in antioxidants and therefore play a very important role in prevention of breast cancer. Those known for having the leanest body mass in the world are the Korean and Japanese people. Their diets are comprised primarily of vegetables, fruits, and seafoods. Korean and Japanese women have a very low incidence of breast cancer. Some studies involving Korean and Japanese women found they experience less depression, fatigue, and bleeding during their menstrual cycles.

Heart Disease

Circulatory problems and heart disease are caused by a higher consumption of fat, calories, and lack of physical exercise. Aging does not bring it about. By reducing fat and calorie intake, you will be better able to control these problems.

High Blood Pressure

Hypertension is responsible for more than a million deaths and strokes each year. It is causes chiefly by high salt intake and obesity. Aging is not responsible. Reducing salt intake and losing weight will aide in controlling this problem.

Digestive Disorders

Several digestive disturbances including constipation, gas, and bloatedness are caused by a high fat diet and a lack of fruits, vegetables, and fiber in the diet. To relieve these problems you will need to reduce the fat in your diet and eat more fruits and vegetables.

Gall Bladder

The gall bladder is a small bag or reservoir for bile acid. Bile acid is produced by the liver and required for the digestion of fat. A high fat diet typically leads to problems related to the gall bladder. The gall bladder is connected to the digestive system by a duct, in order to digest fat in the diet. Sometimes the gall bladder becomes infected, causing extreme pain, and needs to be surgically removed. The solution to this problem is eating a low fat-low protein diet.

PART V
RECIPES FOR HEALTH AND LONGEVITY

29

THE SECRETS OF GOOD HEALTH AND LONGEVITY

Tooshi's Law: "Never give up."

It is a dismal picture that nearly seventy-five (75%) of Americans are overweight and forty (40%) of their children are overweight, that hospitals and doctor's offices are jammed with sick people, and that it is becoming increasingly difficult to secure appointments to see doctors. How did we get to this point when we have the best foods, best exercise equipment, and best medicine in the world? The answer lies in the habits and behavior of the American people. The solution lies in reversing the trend.

For one thing, our portions are too big. We eat too much in one setting. Secondly, we eat too fast. By the time the stomach reports to the brain it is too late to cut the sensation of hunger. We have already consumed a large quantity of food. Thirdly, we eat very little fruit, vegetables and seafood and too much saturated fats. And to make matters worse, we do not exercise on a daily basis. Many Americans do not exercise at all.

Research has been done throughout the world in hopes of revealing the secrets of longevity and good health. These studies show that people who live over ninety years of age without physical and mental problems possess certain characteristics.

- They were physically active all throughout their lives

- They ate mainly seafood, fruits and vegetables

- They ate small meals

- They ate slowly

- They had very little stress

Eat Right to Stay Young:

Eating variety of vegetables is one of the best ways to slow down the aging process. Vegetables with different color provide excellent antioxidants. The colors signify different health benefits. For example, leafy green vegetables contain Vitamin A and Vitamin C, yellows and oranges are high in Vitamin A, purple-colored vegetables such as eggplants are high in Vitamin C. The key to decelerating the aging process lies in eating a variety of antioxidant-rich vegetables. A diet high in antioxidant-rich vegetables will prevent free radicals from building up in the cells. Free radical buildup has a degenerative effect on our DNA and as a result the cells die prematurely. As cells die, the aging process accelerates. Antioxidants prevent free radical buildup inside our cells consequently preventing cell destruction and slowing down the aging process. Anti-oxidant rich foods are related to the glycemic index because they naturally have a low glycemic index.

DR. TOOSHI'S TEN COMMANDMENTS FOR OPTIMAL HEALTH

1. **Throw some fish on the grill.**

   Fish is loaded with omega-3 that helps to lower bad cholesterol and increase good cholesterol.

2. **Add more tomatoes to your diet.**

   Tomatoes contain antioxidants and lycopene,
   Believed to reduce the risk of cardiovascular disease.

3. **Walk Outdoors.**

   Walking 30-45 minutes a day improves the quality of life and reduces tension.

4. **Eat Less.**

   Cut your portions in half.

5. **Eat slowly.**

   It reduces your appetite.

6. **Get a dog.**

   People who own dogs walk more, boosting their health and fitness.

7. **Eat at least four fruits a day.**

   Fruits provide natural sugar, water, minerals, and vitamins. They cleanse your body.

8. **Load up with a variety of vegetables.**

   Vegetables contain chemicals that boost your immune system.

9. **Meditate.**

   Meditation reduces stress and creates harmony between mind and body.

10. **Don't associate with fat people.**

They have a bad influence on your eating habits.

After studying the eating habits of various populations and ethnic groups and their levels of health and disease, I organized a diet to help people to live longer with good health. The following diet regimen can be utilized by anyone seeking to stay young and healthy and free from developing chronic disease.

Breakfast—select one each day

Whole-wheat toast with an egg
A glass of 1% milk with a banana
Low fat yogurt with a fruit
½ cantaloupe
Whole wheat bagel with low-fat, low-salt cheese
Two fruits

Lunch—select one each day

Salad with an apple
Fruit salad
Salad with salmon
Turkey sandwich
Yogurt with fruit

Dinner—select one each day

Fish with vegetables and potato or brown rice
Shrimp with vegetables and brown rice
Grilled turkey with vegetables and potato
Vegetable soup

Snacks—select one

Any fruits, including apple, banana, strawberry, cantaloupe, watermelon, peach, plum, pear
Yogurt with a fruit, low-fat cheese with crackers

Avoid—canned, jarred and bottled foods because they contain excessive salt and chemical additives. Also limit pre-cooked or prepared foods.

Vitamins—certain vitamins are needed for optimal health. Vitamins help us to digest food and to metabolize the foods we eat. Vitamins that help provide energy are B1, B6, and B12. Anti-oxidant vitamins that help prevent cancers are A, C, and E. Vitamins that prevent water retention are B6 and B1. Vitamins E, C, and Selenium promote longevity.

Minerals—three very important minerals should be taken daily. They are potassium, calcium, and magnesium.

When is the best time to take vitamins?

Since the role of vitamins is to digest food and metabolize food, the best time to take vitamins is after dinner, because the dinner meal is mainly a larger meal and consists of a variety of foods. Dinner meals are usually prepared with corn or olive oil. It is necessary to add some oil into the diet in order to gain benefit from taking fat-soluble vitamins. Do not take vitamins on an empty stomach.

NOTE—avoid taking a multi-vitamin. They contain very small amounts of vitamins and do not meet your daily needs.

Selection of good carbohydrates

As previously stated, the main sources of energy for physical activities come from carbohydrates. But not all carbohydrates are the same. Some carbohydrates contain fat, salt, chemicals or additives whereas others are natural and contain no fat, chemicals, and additives. It is vitally important to pay attention in choosing carbohydrate foods, especially to the people who engage in regular exercise.
Good carbohydrates are classified into four groups—vegetables, starches, fruits, legumes
These carbohydrates are called complex carbohydrates and contain vitamins, minerals, fiber, and anti-oxidants.

Vegetables—are all excellent sources of vitamins, minerals, and fiber. They come in a variety of colors—red, green, yellow, and dark colors. Each color provides a specialized anti-oxidant. Some boost the immune system while others slow down the aging process or prevent arthritis.

Starches—are divided into two groups

• Complex

• Non-complex

Complex starches include rice, potatoes, whole wheat bread, rye bread, and corn. These starches contain fiber, vitamins, and minerals.

Non-complex starches include cookies, pie, muffins, pasta, white bread, and cereal. These starches have no fiber, vitamins, or minerals. They contain fat, sugar, salt, and additives.

Fruits—are excellent sources of natural water, sugar, minerals, vitamins, and fiber. They come in a variety of colors. Each fruit contributes a different benefit to the body according to their color. A variety of fruits should be consumed rather than the same fruits every day.

Enzymes—provide very good carbohydrates and also contain very good fat called unsaturated fat, which is good for circulation and lowering high blood cholesterol. Legumes are very high in Vitamin E, contain a variety of minerals such as zinc, magnesium, copper, and calcium, and are very high in fiber. In order to obtain necessary enzymes, a balanced diet should include two servings of fruit, two servings of vegetables, two servings of complex starches, two servings of legumes, and two good proteins—namely poultry and seafood each day.

Your daily diet should include three meals—breakfast, lunch and dinner. All these meals should include some protein, carbohydrates, and fruits.

Snacks—the best snacks are fruits. At least two to three types of fruits should be included your daily diet.

Selection of Good Protein

The functions of protein are:

- Growth of muscles. Bones cannot grow without protein

- Development. Protein helps to maintain development of the body

- Production of enzymes and hormones. Enzymes and hormones protect the body against infection and cancer

Good proteins include foods such as fish, shrimp, chicken, turkey, eggs, and low fat dairy products.

Selection of Good Fat

The human body requires fat to deal with its physiological needs. The body utilizes fat for:

• Protection against radiation

• Production of sex hormones

• Protection of the hair and prevention of dry skin

• Protection of vital organs

• Production of energy

Good fats come from vegetable oil such as corn and olive oil. These fats contain polyunsaturated fat. Polyunsaturated fat prevents high blood cholesterol and contains ingredients, which protect hair from falling out and skin from becoming dry. Saturated fat, which comes from animal sources should be avoided as much as possible. These fats increase blood cholesterol and damage blood vessels. Most heart attacks and strokes are associated with animal fats.

WEIGHT LOSS DIET

Excessive body weight is a most dangerous health problem. Today it is the root of all major diseases including heart disease, cancer, diabetes, stroke, and lack of energy, fatigue, and sleep disturbances. Emotional stress may also be attributed to excessive weight. To lose weight and then to maintain body weight requires a proper and balanced diet program. Essential foods such as complex carbohydrates, good proteins and unsaturated fats, fruits and vegetables must be included in a weight loss regimen. Lack of any of these essential nutrients will have negative effects on your health. Here I have organized a weight loss plan for someone seeking to lose between ten to twenty pounds in one month. If you follow it you will get excellent results. After one month, if you need to lose more than twenty pounds, repeat weeks one through four. After that it is important for you to plan your own diet based on the information learned from my book. All dinner selections can be found in chapter 31.

Week One

Breakfast—select one

A fruit
One slice of toast with jam
An egg, hard-boiled, soft-boiled, or poached

Lunch—select one

Salad with two slices of low-fat cheese
Salad with 3-4 slices of turkey
Salad with a hard-boiled egg

Dinner—select one

Tooshi's Dinner
Fish la Chanta
Egg Omelet

Week Two

Breakfast (select one)
One slice of rye or whole-wheat toast with a slice of low-fat cheese
Oatmeal
Banana

Lunch (select one)
Three slices cheese with an apple
Salad with half-can (3oz) tuna and chopped onion
Salad with an apple

Dinner (select one)
Chicken Cutlet
Stuffed Pepper
Food for Heart with Tooshi's Sauce

Week Three

Breakfast (select one)
Six oz plain low-fat yogurt with raisins or a fruit
Two egg whites
One slice of rye or whole-wheat toast with a slice of low-fat cheese

Lunch (select one)

Salad with 3-4 oz turkey
Salad with two slices low-fat cheese
Four to five oz cottage cheese with a fruit

Dinner (select one)
Mediterranean Dinner
Shrimp Dinner
Meatball Dinner

Week Four

Breakfast (select one)
One slice rye or whole-wheat toast with an egg
A fruit
Half-glass of milk with a banana

Lunch (select one)
Yogurt with a fruit
Tuna (3-4 oz) with chopped onion and a tomato
Half cantaloupe with two tablespoons cottage cheese

Dinner (select one)
Tooshi's Seafood Combo
Tooshi's Soup
Veal Cutlet

Note: Rotate breakfasts, lunches, and dinners each week. Do not eat the same thing every day.
Snack: A fruit after dinner each day, if desired.
Liquids: Water, coffee and tea (1% milk, if you must sweeten choose Equal).
Avoid: Soda, canned, bottled, and jarred foods as all they contain salt, including diet sodas.
Salt: Do not add salt to foods. Use spices or jalapeno instead.
Eating Out: When dining out, select from the following lists.
Breakfast—fruit, toast with an egg, egg omelet
Lunch—salad with grilled chicken, salad with an egg, salad with a fruit.
Dinner—Grilled fish with vegetables, grilled chicken with salad, grilled steak with salad, steamed shrimp with steamed vegetables.

The permanent solution to weight loss

- Reduce the portions

- Eat slowly

- Talk while eating

- Reduce number of snacks

- Eat more fruits, vegetables and seafood

- Reduce red meats, animal fats, soft drinks, cakes, and muffins

- Engage 30 to 45 minutes of cardiovascular activity daily

GLYCEMIC INDEX

How many times have you heard the six golden words: "I am on a new diet?" Even with the countless books available for losing weight the number of overweight people keeps climbing. Nearly 75% of Americans are obese or overweight and childhood obesity has reached epidemic levels. This excess of weight brings with it a host of health problems such as heart disease, cancer, diabetes and high blood pressure. Think of it this way ... if you are consuming mainly processed, chemical-laden, and high fat foods, you are polluting and destroying your body.

Many diets ask you to lower your carbohydrate intake in order to bring about a quick weight loss. However, the weight you lose is mostly water due to the fact that your carbohydrate rich diet caused your system to retain fluid. If you continue to avoid eating carbohydrates, eventually muscle is broken down to produce glucose. Once you give up your diet and return to your former way of eating you regain more fat. So called Yo-Yo dieting causes you to lose more muscle mass over the course of years. You eventually are left with less muscle and more fat and you increase your risk for developing high blood sugar and may become diabetic. To prevent the onset of diabetes it is important to know what our blood sugar response is to the food we eat. It is also important to monitor how much carbohydrate we eat as well as the type of carbohydrates. The use of a system called the Glycemic Index (GI) can help. It is a system of categorizing carbohydrate foods according to their energy output. Foods can be rated as high-, medium- or low-GI. High-GI foods, such as cakes, chocolate, soda, and juice should be avoided as they release energy rapidly into the bloodstream. Low- and medium-GI foods, such as fruits, vegetables, legumes, and nuts, release energy at a steadier rate, which is good for you.

A Glycemic Index can help you select foods to better manage or to prevent diabetes. It is not related to lowering carbohydrates foods or eliminating them in the diet, rather selecting low glycemic foods.

GLYCEMIC TABLE

The Glycemic Index is arranged from zero to one hundred, with zero being lowest and one hundred being highest. The foods with a lower glycemic index are useful for controlling blood sugar. The richest sources of carbohydrates include: bread, pasta, potatoes, baked goods, breakfast cereals, and potato products. Selecting low glycemic index foods will significantly lower your blood sugar and prevent diabetes. Low glycemic foods include: breads (made from whole grain or stone-ground flour); rice (brown rice, imported Japanese or long-grain white rice); grains (barley, buckwheat, corn); legumes (beans, chickpeas, lentils); cereals (Bran, Grapenuts, Oatbran, Special K); crackers (stone ground wheat thins); fruits (apples, pears, citrus fruits); vegetables (cherries, plums, peaches). Vegetables generally help lower blood sugar due to their low glycemic index. Canned vegetables, fruits, and legumes are good for controlling blood sugar; however, they are also very high in salt and added sugars. Therefore, you should rinse them thoroughly to reduce the salt and sugar content before eating them.

Low Glycemic Foods for Diabetics

- Fruits: Apple, peach, pear, plum, cherries and oranges

- Bread: Stone ground wheat

- Rice: Uncle Ben's converted brown rice

- Potatoes: yams, sweet potatoes

- Legumes: all beans, chickpeas

- Crackers: stone ground wheat thins

- Vegetables: all green leafy varieties

However, diabetics should avoid the following

Sugar—is a major source of free radical and causes skin problems.

Salt—high salt intake causes water retention and high blood pressure.

Alcohol—robs the body from vitamins and causes liver problems.

Coffee—coffee is a stimulant and it increases pulse, blood pressure, and causes hypoglycemia. More than two cups a day creates health problems.

Water—watch your water intake. Do not drink more than five glasses of water. If you are very thirsty check your diet. Maybe you are taking too much salt.

30

QUESTIONS and ANSWERS

Why do I often get bloated after eating and develop embarrassing flatulence?

Bloating indicates a digestive problem and you may be eating foods high in fat and sugar. The symptoms are a distended abdomen, abdominal pain, and flatulence. The solution lies in lowering the fat content in your diet by avoiding whole milk dairy products, fried foods, and desserts. Sugar is a fundamental piece of the fermentation process in the digestive tract, especially when it is combined with flour and yeast products. For those experiencing both bloatedness and gas; they may have a problem digesting fat and should have their gall bladder checked. Eating slowly, drinking water with meals, and reducing sugar generally reduces bloatedness.

I often suffer from constipation. Is it something I ate?

Anything that prolongs the transit time of food to move through the bowels likely leads to constipation. Avoiding dressings, mayonnaise, sauces, and fried foods and increasing fresh fruits and vegetables in your diet may alleviate the problem. Laxatives are not a solution. Constipation is caused by a low fiber diet, not drinking enough water, lack of physical exercise, and emotional stress.

I'm cranky and have no energy. Might I be allergic to certain foods?

Chances are that you may have low blood sugar. Check first with your doctor to rule out hypoglycemia and try avoiding cake, cookies, ice cream, and non-complex carbohydrate foods. So-called food allergies are generally attributed to chemical preservatives and food colorings. Avoid jarred, canned, boxed and bagged foods. Another rule of thumb is to avoid foods with a high shelf life. For example, canned soups, tuna, potato chips, and ketchup all have a high shelf life of approximately one year. Increasing fresh and frozen vegetables is a better option to canned and jarred foods.

Why do I wake up at night with heartburn?

Your dinner may contain too much fat. Try to reduce fat intake. It may help to raise the head part of your bed six inches higher. Wood blocks or bricks that elevate the headboard legs of the bed two to six inches are more effective than extra pillows.

I hate to eat lunch at work because I feel tired and sluggish shortly afterward.

You are likely eating carbohydrate rich foods. Try eating citrus fruits such as an orange, grapefruit, or plum with a sandwich for lunch.

I always seem to catch colds or unable to get off antibiotics. Is my immune system working?

We must take steps to address the factors that reduce immune function, namely stress, free radicals, and chemical toxins. Stress, free radicals, and chemical toxins leave you prone to colds, flu and other bacterial ailments. By increasing vitamins A, C and the mineral zinc, can help your body cope with the negative effects of stress and boost the lymphatic system, which manufactures and stores white blood cells. In addition, selenium is a powerful mineral antioxidant. Selenium rich foods include mushrooms, legumes and sunflower seeds. Selenium also plays a vital role is slowing down the aging process. Garlic has a long history of being an immune booster. That is why garlic is an ingredient in most of my recipes. Adding yogurt to your diet helps to restore good bacteria, improving digestion and absorption of immune boosting nutrients.

Why do I feel thirsty and get up in the middle of the night to go to the bathroom?

Feeling thirsty is symptomatic of high blood sugar. Check your blood sugar.

Thirst also occurs from taking too much sodium in your diet. Sources include jarred, canned or bottled foods as well as snack foods such as potato chips and pretzels.

Why do I have no energy when I get up in the morning?

You may be eating carbohydrate rich/starchy foods after dinner. Avoid snack foods, ice cream, cakes and cookies. Try fruit instead. Starchy foods raise blood sugar, which stimulates insulin production. Insulin causes your blood sugar to go down below normal levels. Avoid carbohydrate rich and starchy foods altogether before bedtime usually alleviates this problem.

I get tired most afternoons around one or two o'clock. What causes that?

One reason is that by afternoon, your blood sugar drops as a result of eating too much carbohydrate foods for breakfast. Eating a fruit when fatigue occurs usually remedies the problem. The other reason pertains to diabetics, who may be taking too much insulin and need to consult their doctor. Too much insulin lowers the blood sugar and makes you feel tired. Take a half glass of orange juice when feeling lightheaded. If you have been diagnosed as having low blood sugar, then eating 3-4 small meals per day and lowering carbohydrates and increasing protein is the best remedy to fatigue. For example, a turkey sandwich on toast with lettuce, tomato, and onion around 3:00 pm is an effective way to manage fatigue caused by low blood sugar.

Why do I get diarrhea once in awhile?

You may have gotten bacteria from the food you ate. The most common sources of bacteria in food are from salad bars without proper temperature control or that are not routinely replaced and chicken and seafood not properly cooked. The solution is to cook all meats well at home and to eat out in clean and air conditioned restaurants. Salad bars should be set over ice or look crisp and fresh.

What is the cause of acid reflux? I often get it after eating.

Acid reflux or GERD is caused by overeating fatty foods such as fried foods, snack foods baked in oils, regular dairy products, salad dressings, and artificial dairy creamers. Frequent heartburn is the most common symptom of GERD and usually occurs after eating. Damage to the esophagus may occur as a result of gastric acid backing up from the stomach. Eating smaller meals, losing weight, reducing spicy and high fat foods, and avoiding tight clothing generally alleviates the symptoms of GERD.

I have a problem sleeping. What is keeping me awake all night?

Periodic difficulty in sleeping may come from water retention. Water retention is caused by high salt intake. High salt intake disturbs the electrolyte balance and causes nervous tension. Nervous tension disrupts sleeping. To remedy, reduce salt intake.

A more chronic inability to sleep is called insomnia. Insomnia is caused by emotional stress but can also be related to a high intake of noncomplex carbohydrate foods before bedtime. The remedy is to get involved with meditation and exercise and by avoiding starchy foods before bedtime. Eating or working too late and eating high-GI foods may contribute to persistent sleeplessness. Eating low-GI foods at dinner tends to stabilize blood sugar, ensuring a sounder night's sleep.

I generally feel tired and have no energy. Why?

A deficiency in vitamins and minerals in the diet, particularly a lack of iron and potassium, may cause lack of energy. Water retention caused by excess salt intake, high blood sugar (hyperglycemia), or low blood sugar (hypoglycemia) are other factors responsible for lack of energy. A blood test will reveal if your blood sugar is too high or too low. One of the dangers of prolonged lack of energy is mood swings and depression. Studies have revealed that diet and lifestyle are the major factors influencing depression or mood swings. A tired nervous system may leave you susceptible to depression or mood swings. The mind-body link is a well-documented phenomenon.

I am always hungry. What causes that?

You are eating too many simple carbohydrates that rapidly raise blood sugar very high. The body's response is to release a large amount of insulin, which brings blood sugar down below the normal range. This is what triggers your hunger shortly after eating carbohydrate rich foods. The solution is portion control and in avoiding simple carbohydrates such as donuts, bagels, cake, pie, cookies. In the meantime have your blood sugar tested.

I have dry skin. What causes it?

Dry skin comes from a deficiency of iron. Eating foods high in iron such as liver, eggs, and raisins and cooking in corn oil are one solution. Supplementing the diet with Iron and vitamin C is another solution.

31

DR. TOOSHI'S RECIPES

These recipes are unique, unlike other recipes you have tried. They do not contain any saturated fats, making them very low fat, yet delicious. There are no chemical preservatives or additives in the ingredients. Salt is not necessary to improve the natural flavors. All the recipes are naturally low-calorie (350-400 calories) and can serve two people. What makes my recipes so unique is that I have combined both low-fat and high-fiber ingredients and still permit you to select a variety of vegetables. Most diet recipes are high-protein/low-fiber or high-fiber/high-saturated fat. My recipes are easy to prepare, healthy, and time-tested, not more than 30-minutes start to finish. An added bonus is my recipes are good for people who have high blood pressure, high cholesterol, high blood sugar, and problems with their digestive system such as constipation, gas, bloatedness, or acid reflux. They are excellent meal plans for anyone seeking to lose weight.

Baked Veal Cutlet

Ingredients:

Six ounces veal cutlet
One or two tomatoes
Five mushrooms
Select broccoli, cabbage or spinach
One fresh lemon
One-teaspoon corn or olive oil
Spices you like (no salt)

Directions:

Pre-heat oven to 450
Place veal cutlet onto a sheet of aluminum foil with vegetables around the cutlet
Add corn or olive oil
Add seasonings
Slice lemon and place over the veal cutlet
Wrap tightly
Cook 20-25 minutes and serve

Chicken Cutlet

Ingredients:

Six ounces chicken cutlet
Three tablespoons orange juice
Spices: onion and garlic powder, red or black pepper
Select any of the following vegetables:

Cabbage	Peppers	Broccoli
Cauliflower	Asparagus	Zucchini

Directions:

Place the chicken cutlet in a baking dish
Combine spices and orange juice in a mixing bowl
Brush half the mixture over the cutlet and cook in the oven at 400 degrees for 10-12 minutes

Turn cutlet over, brush remaining mixture on the other side, and then add vegetables to the baking dish.
Return to the oven. Cook another 10-12 minutes and serve

Chicken La Supreme

Ingredients:

Six oz chicken cutlet
¼ cup of wine
Two tablespoons grated cheese
Half cup each mushroom, tomato, and broccoli
Onion and garlic powder

Directions:

Pre-heat oven to 350 degrees
Place chicken cutlet in center of a baking dish
Add wine and sprinkle grated cheese and spices over the chicken
Cover and bake 15-18 minutes
Serve with steamed vegetables
Note: You may substitute other vegetables according to your taste

Diabetic Vegetables

Ingredients:

Kidney Beans	Tablespoon of corn
Lentils	½ cup water
Cabbage	Spices-onion & garlic powder
Broccoli	Fresh garlic
Onion	

Directions:

Soak dry kidney beans and lentils at least 8 hours before cooking
Cook the beans 5-10 minutes in ½ cup of water

Chop all vegetables. Add to the beans
Cook 5-8 minutes and serve with chicken or fish
Canned kidney beans and lentils may be substituted. Drain and rinse

Egg Omelet

Ingredients:

Three tomatoes
Six mushrooms
One fresh garlic
One-teaspoon corn oil
Two eggs
Spices you like (no salts)
One tablespoon grated cheese

Directions:

Add one-tablespoon corn oil to a frying pan
Chop and add all vegetables and spices
Cover and cook over medium heat 6-8 minutes or until all juice comes out of tomatoes
Uncover, add two eggs, and mix well
Cover and cook another 2-3 minutes and serve

Fish La Chanta

Ingredients:

Six ounces flounder
Three tomatoes
One fresh garlic
Six tomatoes
One-teaspoon corn oil
¼ cup water
Spices: onion powder, garlic powder, oregano

Directions:

Add one-teaspoon corn oil to a frying pan with ¼ cup water

Heat the pan before adding flounder and seasonings
Cover and cook six minutes
Remove lid and let water evaporate
Add chopped vegetables to the flounder
Cover and cook 6-8 minutes and serve

Food for Heart

Ingredients:

4-6 ounces salmon
Tooshi's Sauce
Fresh lemon

Directions:

Bake the salmon in oven or on the grill
Prepare Tooshi's Sauce
Serve the salmon over Tooshi's Sauce with fresh lemon slices

French Delight

Ingredients:

Six ounces fish
One onion
One whole garlic
Eight mushrooms
Two tomatoes
½ zucchini
¼ eggplant
½ tablespoon corn or olive oil

Directions:

Chop all vegetables except tomatoes and place in a wok or skillet
Add oil and mix well
Cover wok or skillet and cook until the onions are browned
Lower the heat. Place fish on top of the vegetables
Chop and add tomatoes over the fish. Do not mix.

Cover and cook over medium heat 12-15 minutes and serve with fresh lemon

Grilled Eggplant

Ingredients:

One medium eggplant
Two plum tomatoes
*Grated cheese or four slices Alpine Lace cheese
Spices you like

Directions:

1. Slice the eggplant in half lengthwise
2. Slice the plum tomatoes lengthwise and place over the top of each eggplant half
3. Add grated cheese over the tomatoes
4. Bake for 20 minutes at 400 degrees and serve
*If you prefer to use Alpine Lace cheese, do not add grated cheese (step 3). Follow steps 1,2, and 4. Turn oven off. Add Alpine lace cheese on top of tomatoes, return to oven and let sit for one minute, and then serve.

Grilled Seafood Combo

Ingredients:

Three ounces scallops
Three ounces shrimp
Two teaspoons corn oil
Spices: onion powder, garlic powder, oregano

Directions:

Place shrimp and scallops onto aluminum foil. Add corn oil and spices
Wrap foil around the seafood
Bake in oven or on grill for 15 minutes at 400 degrees
Serve with Tooshi's Sauce

Hudson Salad Dressing

Ingredients:

Unlimited vinegar or Balsamic vinegar
Half-tablespoon corn or olive oil
1/3 cup lemon juice
Onion and garlic powder
Teaspoon of pepper and basil
Dash of mustard, if desired

Directions:

Combine all ingredients in a container
Shake well and chill
Add to salad
Add more vinegar or Balsamic vinegar if desired

Hudson Shish-Ka-Bab

Ingredients:

Six ounces chicken cutlet
Two tomatoes
Six mushrooms
One onion
¼ cup wine
Spices: onion and garlic powder, oregano and pepper

Directions:

Cut chicken into cubes
Cut vegetables into wedges
Arrange chicken, tomato, mushroom, and onion alternately onto a spear
Add spices and sprinkle with wine
Cook in the oven or grill until meat is roasted

La Fish

Ingredients:

Six ounces flounder
½ cup dry wine
Fresh crushed garlic
One medium tomato
One diced onion
Four mushrooms
Chopped parsley
Half tablespoon lemon juice

Directions:

Add ¼ cup wine to a frying pan and bring to a boil
Add flounder, onion, garlic and ½ tablespoon lemon juice
Cover pan and sauté fish on both sides a total of eight minutes
Add mushroom, tomato and parsley
Cook another 6-8 minutes and serve

Legume Vegetarian II

Ingredients:

Variety of dry beans
Tomatoes
Mushrooms
Three ounces low fat cheese
Seasonings

Directions:

Soak the beans 5-6 hours prior to cooking
Add water and boil 6-8 minutes
Prepare Tooshi's Sauce adding three ounces low-fat cheese
Mix ingredients well. Drain excess water from beans
Add Tooshi's Sauce to the beans
Simmer five minutes and serve
Note: If you prefer to use canned beans, rinse first to remove salt

Liver La France

Ingredients:

Six ounces chicken liver or beef liver
One onion
Four mushrooms
One whole garlic
Two tomatoes
One-tablespoon corn oil or olive oil
Spices

Directions:

Chop the onion; add to a frying pan with one-tablespoon oil
Slice beef liver into small cubes and add to chopped onion. Mix well
Cover and cook 10 minutes over high heat or until mixture becomes browned
Chop mushroom, garlic and tomatoes. Add to the frying pan. Mix well
Cover and cook another 10 minutes or until tomatoes become a sauce
Mix well and serve
Note: If tomatoes are too watery, remove lid and continue to simmer until water
evaporates

Mediterranean Delight

Ingredients:

Six ounces chicken cutlet
One onion
One whole garlic
Eight mushrooms
Two tomatoes
Half zucchini
¼ eggplant
Half-tablespoon corn or olive oil

Directions:

Chop all vegetables except tomatoes and place in a wok or skillet
Add oil. Mix well

Cover and cook until onions are brown
Lower the heat
Cut chicken into strips and place on top of the vegetables
Chop and add tomatoes over the cutlets. Do not mix
Cover and cook over medium heat12-15 minutes
Serve with fresh lemon wedges

Oriental Supreme

Ingredients:

Half-cup dry white rice
Half zucchini
Two tomatoes
Five mushrooms
¼ eggplant
One-teaspoon corn or olive oil
Spices

Directions:

Empty half cup of rice into a saucepan
Add water so that water is one inch above the rice
Cover and cook over high heat until rice boils
Lower to medium heat. Continue cooking ten minutes.
Remove the lid and set pan in shallow water to cool to prevent rice from sticking to the bottom of the pan
In another saucepan cut and add all the vegetables with one cup of water and teaspoon oil.
Add spices. Boil five minutes and serve over rice

Pe-Co Vegetarian Mix

Ingredients:

Half-cup peas and corn combined
¼ cup red kidney beans
¼ cup chickpeas
Four mushrooms

Two tomatoes
One onion
One pepper
One zucchini
Half-cup cabbage
Four slices low fat cheese

Directions:

Cut all vegetables. Place into a wok
Cover and cook 15 minutes on high heat
Add cheese to the top of the vegetables
Continue to cook another five minutes and serve
Note: Should you prefer to bake this recipe, choose a Pyrex baking dish
And set oven to 400 degrees. Follow same cooking steps

Roasted Chicken

Ingredients:

Chicken cutlet
One lemon or orange
Corn or olive oil

Directions:

Slice the cutlet lengthwise not more than one inch thick
Rub oil onto a sheet of aluminum foil and place unto a baking tray
Arrange the chicken on the foil. Rub a small amount of oil on top of the cutlets
so that both sides are coated
Add lemon or orange slices over the cutlets and bake at 400 degrees for 15-20
minutes or until lightly roasted
Serve with Tooshi's Sauce or mixed vegetables

Scallops Du Pan

Ingredients:

Six ounces scallops
¼ cup water

One-teaspoon corn or olive oil
One cup chopped mushroom
Two tomatoes
One fresh garlic
One fresh lemon
One cup chopped spinach
Spices

Directions:

Mix ¼ cup water with teaspoon oil to a preheated frying pan. Add spices and bring to a boil
Lower the flame, add scallops, and cook with lid on for 8-10 minutes
Remove lid. Continue cooking until all water evaporates
Add chopped mushroom, tomato, and garlic. Cover and cook another 6-8 minutes and serve with fresh lemon

Shrimp Dinner

Ingredients:

Six medium shrimp
Two fresh tomatoes
One fresh garlic
Six mushrooms
One-teaspoon corn or olive oil
¼ cup water
Spices

Directions:

Add teaspoon oil and ¼ cup water to frying pan. Add seasonings and bring to a boil
Add shrimp
Cover and cook 5-6 minutes on high
Remove cover and continue cooking until all water evaporates
Chop and add tomatoes, then mushroom and garlic. Lower the heat and continue cooking 3-4 minutes and serve

Shrimp Salad Delight

Ingredients:

Six shrimp	Romaine lettuce
One tomato	Half cucumber
Half green pepper	Lemon and vinegar
Four radish	Spices or a dash of mustard

Directions:

Boil the shrimp for 2-3 minutes on high
Remove from pan and marinate in refrigerator with lemon, vinegar and spices
When ready, slice shrimp in half and mix with prepared salad. Add marinate mixture. Toss well and serve

Stuffed Chicken Cutlet

Ingredients:

4-6 ounces chicken cutlet sliced thinly
½ cup chopped spinach
½ cup chopped onion
½ chopped scallions
¼ cup dry white wine or lemon juice
½ teaspoon paprika
One carrot
1 cup string beans
1 teaspoon corn or olive oil

Directions:

Mix all chopped vegetables with oil and spread them over each thin slice of cutlet
Roll up and fasten with toothpicks
Place cutlets onto aluminum foil
Pour wine or lemon juice over them
Slice carrots and beans. Arrange them around the cutlets. Sprinkle with paprika
Cover with foil and bake at 350 degrees for 25 minutes and serve

Stuffed Flounder

Ingredients:

4 filet of flounder
1 cup chopped spinach
1 cup chopped scallion
1 tablespoon lemon juice
¼ cup dry white wine or water
½ teaspoon paprika

Directions:

Spread chopped spinach, scallion, and onion over each flounder fillet
Roll up and fasten with toothpicks. Place fish in a non-stick baking dish or line with foil
Pour wine and lemon juice over the fillets
Sprinkle with paprika and bake at 350 degrees for 25 minutes and serve

Stuffed Peppers

Ingredients:

2 ounces ground beef
½ chopped onion
2chopped mushrooms
½ of one garlic
1 teaspoon grated cheese
1 tomato
2 large green peppers

Directions:

Cook chop meat in a saucepan with ½ cup of water for 8-10 minutes.
Drain well and set aside
Chop and mix all vegetables
Add to chop meat. Mix well and cook 6-7 minutes over medium heat
Slice the caps off the peppers and stuff bottoms with chop meat and vegetable mixture

Secure tops with toothpicks
Cover and cook in the oven at 350 degrees for 8-10 minutes then serve

Tooshi's Combo

Ingredients:

4-6 ounces lean beef
½ cup each of broccoli, mushroom, spinach and string beans
1 fresh garlic
3-4 tablespoons Tooshi's Sauce
Spices

Directions:

Slice beef into thin strips. Arrange onto sheet of aluminum foil
Place vegetables around the beef strips
Add 3-4 tablespoons Tooshi's Sauce
Bake in the oven at 350 degrees for 20 minutes and then serve

Tooshi's Dinner

Ingredients:

Select six to eight ounces of the following

Shrimp	Turkey cutlet	Chicken Liver
Scallops	Chicken cutlet	

2 tomatoes
1 whole garlic
1 medium onion
Mushrooms and bean sprouts
Spices
Select either ½ cup wine or ¼ cup water with 1/2tablespoon corn or olive oil

Directions:

Preheat a frying pan for one minute

Add your selection of wine or water and oil along with you choice of meat to the pan

Note: poultry should be chopped into bite-sized pieces

Cover and cook 8-10 minutes over medium-high heat

Remove lid, mix well, and add spices

Continue to cook with lid off until all water evaporates and the meat or seafood becomes browned

Chop and add all vegetables, cover and simmer over medium to low heat another 6-8 minutes and serve

Tooshi's Meatball Dinner

Ingredients:

Four to six ounces low fat chopped turkey or beef

Two ounces bread crumbs

One-half onion

Directions:

Chop the onion well

Mix onion, breadcrumbs and chopped turkey or beef together

Form into three meatballs

Baked the meatballs at 375 for twenty minutes

Serve with Tooshi's Sauce

Tooshi's Sauce

Ingredients:

2 tomatoes

1 fresh garlic

5 mushrooms

1 teaspoon corn or olive oil

Spices

1 tablespoon grated cheese

Directions:

Preheat a frying pan for one minute

Add chopped tomatoes and oil
Cover and cook 5 minutes over medium heat or until all the juice comes out of the tomatoes
Add cheese and seasonings. Chop mushrooms and garlic and add to the tomatoes
Mix well. Cover and cook another 5 minutes and serve with main meal

Tooshi's Soup

Ingredients:

Select either 6-8 ounces of chicken cutlet, turkey cutlet or chicken liver
Celery, carrot, cabbage, tomato, onion, scallion, Swiss chard or any other fresh vegetable
½ tablespoon corn or olive oil
Barley and lentils (1/4 cup per person total)
Spices

Directions:

Boil the cutlets or liver along with barley and lentils in 2 cups of water and ½ tablespoon oil for ten minutes in a deep Teflon pan, covered, over high heat
Chop the vegetables and add to the mixture. Continue boiling another 8-10 minutes
Soup will be ready to serve with fresh lemon squeezed to taste

Vegetarian Dinner

Ingredients:

½ zucchini
2 tomatoes
1 cup each chopped spinach, broccoli, string beans, and mushrooms
1 whole garlic
2 slices low-fat cheese
½ cup water
½ tablespoon corn or olive oil
Spices

Directions:

Chop all vegetables. Add to deep frying pan or soup pot
Add water and oil
Cover and cook 8 minutes over medium to high heat
Reduce heat, mix well, and drain excess water
Add seasonings, and simmer another 5 minutes
Arrange vegetables on dinner plate. Add two slices of low-fat cheese as a topping
Once cheese has melted, serve

32

REFERENCES

Books

Arnot, Bob Dr., <u>The Breast Cancer Prevention Diet</u>. New York: Little, Brown and Company, 1999.

Clark, Carolyn Chambers, <u>Living Well With Menopause</u>. New York: Harper-Colins Publishers, 2005.

Cooper, K.H., <u>The Aerobics Program for Total Well-Being</u>. New York: Bantam Books, 1983.

Mayer, J. <u>Overweight: Causes, Cost and Control</u>. Englewood Cliffs, N.J.: Prentice-Hall, 1968.

Miller, David and Allen, Earl T., <u>Fitness: A Lifetime Commitment</u>. New York: MacMillan, 1990.

Northrup, C., <u>Woman's Bodies, Woman's Wisdom</u>. New York: Bantam Books, 1994.

Sheldon, W., Stevens, S.S., and Tucker, W.B., <u>The Varieties of Human Physique</u>. Darien, Conn.: Hafner, 1970.

Tooshi, Alan M., <u>Dr. Tooshi's High Fiber Diet, A Revolutionary Diet That Will Help</u>

<u>You to Lose Weight, Prevent Cancer, Heart Disease, and Digestive Disorders</u>. Writer's Showcase, Lincoln, NE, 2000.

Articles & Periodicals

Abraham, W.M., "Factors in delayed muscle soreness." Medicine and Science in Sports 9 (1): 11-20, 1977.

Albertazzi, P., Pansini, F., Bonaccorsi, G., et al. "The effect of dietary soy supplementation on hot flashes." Obstretrics and Gynecology, 91: 6-11, 1998.

American College of Physicians. "Position statement: Eating disorders: Anorexia nervosa and bulimia." Philadelphia: American College of Physicians, 1986.

American College of Sports Medicine. Opinion statement: Participation of the female athlete in long distance running. Medicine and Science in Sports 11 (4): 9, 1979.

Barone, J., and Barnett, R. "Eat Smart." American Health Magazine 6 (2): 64-69, 1987.

Blair, S.N., "Physical activity leads to fitness and pays off." The Physician and Sportsmedicine 13 (3): 153-157, 1985.

Bic, Z, Blix, G.G., Hopp, H.P., Leslie, F.M., and Schell, M.J. "The influence of a low-fat diet on incidence and severity of migraine headaches." Journal of Woman's Health Gender Based Medicine, pp. 623-630, June 1999.

Borgen, J.S., and Cohen, C.B., "Eating disorders among female athletes." The physician and Sportsmedicine 15 (2): 89-90, 90-95, 1987.

Burkitt, D.P., "The link between low-fiber diets and diseases." Readings in health, 80/81. Guilford, Conn.: Dushkin Publishing Group, 1980.

Burr, M.L. and. Sweetman, P.M, "Vegetarianism, dietary fiber, and mortality." American Journal of Clinical Nutrition 36: 173, 1982.

Byers, T., Rock, C., and K., Hamilton, "Dietary changes after breast cancer." Cancer Practice 5, no. 5. 1997.

Caspersen, C.J., Physical inactivity and coronary heart disease. The Physician and Sportsmedicine. 15 (11): 43-44, 1987.

Castelli, W.P., and Griffin, G.C., How to help patients cut down on saturated fat. Postgraduate medicine 84 (3): 44-56, 1988.

Chalmers, T.C., "Effects of ascorbic acid on the common cold." American Journal of Medicine 58: 532-536, 1975.

Chandler, C.A, and Marston, R.M., "Fat in the U.S. Diet." Nutrition Program News (USDA publication) May/August 1976.

"Choline and lecithin in the treatment of neurologic disorders," Nutrition and the MD, April 1980.

Chopra, J.G., Forbes, A.L., and Habicht, J.P., "Protein in the U.S. Diet." Journal of the American Dietetic Association 72: 253-258, 1978.

Conner-Greene, P.A., "An educational group treatment program for bulimia." Journal of American College Health 35 (3): 229-231, 1987.

Costill, D.L., and Saltin, B. "Factors limiting gastric emptying during rest and exercise." Journal of Applied Physiology 37 (5): 679-683, 1974.

Dailey, R.K., Neale, A.V., Northrup, J., West, P., and Schwartz, K.L. "Herbal product use and menopause symptom relief in primary care patients: a MetroNet study." Journal of Woman's Health, pp. 633-641, September 2003.

Daniels, J., Fitts, R., and Sheehan, G. "Conditioning for distance running." New York: John Wiley and Sons, 1978.

DeLorne, T.L. "Restoration of muscle power by heavy resistance exercise." Archives of Physical Medicine 27: 645-667, 1945.

Deutsch, C.H., "Fast-food chains wage stomach wars." N.Y. Times Service in Wilmington Star News, March 13, 1988, Wilmington, N.C.

Ernst, N. et al, "The association of plasma high density lipoprotein cholesterol with dietary intake and alcohol consumption." Circulation 62 (suppl. 4): 41-52, 1980.

Fast-food chains. Consumer Report 44: 508-513, 1979.

"Folate and B6 from food or supplements shown to reduce heart disease risk." February 9, 2004. http://www.ProHealthNetwork.com.

Gorbach, Sherwood L. "Diet and the excretion and enterohepatic cycling of estrogens." Preventive Medicine 16: 525-531, 1987.

Grant, W.B. "The role of milk and sugar in heart disease." American Journal of Natural Medicine 5(9): 19-23; 1998.

Halterman, J.S., Kaczorowski, J.M., Aligne, C.A., et al. "Iron deficiency and cognitive achievement among school-aged children and adolescents in the United States." Pediatrics 107: 1381-1386; 2001.

Harris, W.S., "Health effects of omega-3 fatty acids." Contemporary Nutrition 10 (8): 1-2, 1985.

Havel, R.J., "High-density lipoproteins, cholesterol transport, and coronary heart disease." Circulation 60 (1): 1-3, 1979.

Haycock, C.E., and Gillette, J. "Susceptibility of women athletes to injury." Journal of the American Medical Association 236:163-164, 1976.

Herbert, V.D., "Megavitamin Therapy." Contemporary Nutrition 2 (October 1977).

Herzog, D.B., and Copeeland, P.M. "Eating disorders." The New England Journal of Medicine 313 (5): 295-303, 1985.

Jackson, A.S., and Pollock, M.L., "Practical assessment of body composition." The Physician and Sportsmedicine 13 (5): 76, 78-80, 82-90, 1985.

Jepson, R., Mihaljevic, L., and Craig, J. "Cranberries for preventing urinary tract infection." Cochrane Database System Review 2:2, 2004.

Johnson, K. "Exercise improves libido in menopausal women." Clinical Psychiatry News, p. 50, December 2003 .

Joint National Committee on Detection, Evaluation and Treatment of High Blood Pressure, 1980 Report, NIH publication no.81-1088 (Washington C.C. Government Printing Office, 1980).

Joseph, J.J., and Bena, L.L., "Cholesterol reduction—a long term intense exercise program." Journal of Sports Medicine and Physical Fitness 17 (2): 163-168, 1977.

Kaminsky, L. "Walk to keep the holiday pounds off." Ball State University News Release, December 9, 2003. http://www.beu.edu/news.

Kennedy, A.R., "The evidence for soybean products as cancer preventive agents." Journal of Nutrition 125, no. 3: 733S-743S, 1995.

Kennedy, K.I., "Effects of breast-feeding on woman's health." Internal Journal of Gynecology and Obstetrics 47: S11-S20, 1994.

Kemmler, W., Lauber,D., Weineck,J., Kalender,W., et al. "Benefits of 2 years of intense exercise on bone density, physical fitness, and blood lipids in early postmenopausal osteopenic women: results of the Erlangen Fitness Osteoporosis Prevention Study (EFOPS)." Archives of Internal Medicine 164 (10): 1084-1091; 2004.

Key, T.J., Allen, N.E., Spencer, E.A., and Travis, R.C. "Nutrition and breast cancer." Breast 12 (6): 412-416; 2003.

Kolata, G., Value of low-sodium diets questioned (research news), Science 216

(1982): 38-39.

Konishi and S.L. Harrison, "Vitamin D for adults," Journal of Nutrition Education 11: 120-122, 1979.

LaPorte, R.E. "Cardiovascular fitness: Is it really necessary?" The Physician and Sportsmedicine 13 (3): 145-150, 1985.

Lee, K.A., et al. "Folate, iron and restless legs syndrome." Journal of Woman's Health and Gender-Based Medicine 10 (4): 335-431.

Leibel, R.L., et al., "Dieting: your metabolism fights weight loss." New England Journal of Medicine, March 1995, pp. 621-624.

Liu, J., Burdette, J.E., Xu, H., Gu, C., van Breemen, R.B., et al. "Evaluation of estrogenic activity of plant extracts for the potential treatment of menopausal symptoms." Journal of Agricultural and Food Chemistry, pp. 2427-2479, May 2001.

M. Jacobson and B.F. Liebman, "Dietary sodium and the risk of hypertension," Nutrition Reviews 42: 205-213, 1984.

Mann, D., "Soy products, ginseng may lower breast cancer risk." Medical Tribune, p.33. November 27, 1997.

McCunny, R.J., "Fitness, heart disease and high-density lipoproteins: A look at the relationships." The Physician and Sportsmedicine 15 (2): 67-79, 1987.

Marx, J.L.,"The HDL: The good cholesterol carriers?" Science, 205: 677-679, 1979.

Neal, K.G. "Knowledge of health series." Long Beach, Ca.: ELOT Publishing, 1975.

Newman, L., "More "Salt" talks: Diet and hypertension." Journal of the American Medical Association, 248:2949-2951, 1982.

Northrup, C., "Menopause." Complementary and Alternative Therapies in Primary Care 24 (4): 921-946, 1998.

Osganian, S.K., Stampfer, M.J., Rimm, E., Spiegelman, D, Hu, F.B., Manson, J.E., and Willett, W.C. "Vitamin C and risk of coronary heart disease in women." Journal of the American College of Cardiology, pp. 246-252, July 16, 2003.

Paffenbarger, R.S., et al. "Physical activity, all-cause mortality, and longevity of college alumni." New England Journal of Medicine 314 (10): 605-613, 1986.

Pearson, D. "Weight training helps the body look younger." University Communications, Muncie, IN. June 2004. http://www.bsu.edu/newsucomm@bsu.edu.

Potischman, N., Coates, R.J., Swanson, C.A., Carroll, R.J., et al. "Increased risk of early-stage breast cancer related to consumption of sweet foods among women less than age 48 in the Unites States." Cancer Causes and Control 13 (10): 937-946.

Prentice, Ross, "Dietary fat reduction and plasma estradiol concentration in healthy post-menopausal women." Journal of the National Cancer Institute 82, no. 2, 1990.

Sagon, C. Many popular diets lack nutrition needs. Dallas Times Herald in The greenvilkle News, Greenville, S.C., February 22, 1984.

Satoh, T., Sakurai, I, Miyagi,K., and Hohshaku, Y. "Walking exercise and improved neuropsychological functioning in elderly patients with cardiac disease." Journal of Internal Medicine 238 (5): 423-428; 1995.

Shimizu, H., Serum estrogen levels in Postmenopausal women: comparison of American whites and Japanese in Japan, British Journal of Cancer 61: 421-433, 1990.

Su, K.P., Huang, S.Y., Chiu, C.C., and Shen, W.W. "Omega-3 fatty acids in major depressive disorder." European Neuropharmacology 13 (4): 261-271; 2003.

"The health benefits of exercise" (Part 2 of 2). The Physician and Sportsmedicine 15 (11): 121-131, 1987.

Tooshi, A. "Effects of three different durations of endurance exercise upon serum cholesterol in middle-aged men." Doctoral dissertation, University of Illinois, 1970. Published in Medicine and Science in Sports, Vol. 1, 1971.

Tooshi, A. "Effects of endurance jogging program on cardiovascular system and body composition in middle-aged women." National Convention of the American Association for Health, Physical Education, and Recreation, Minneapolis, Minnesota, April 1973.

Tuomainen, T.P., Punnonen, K., Nyyssonene, K.I., and Salonen, J.T. "Association between body iron stores and the risk of acute myocartdial infarction in men." Circulation 97 (15): 1461-1446; 1998.

"Vitamin B12 Deficiency in the breast-fed infant of a strict vegetarian." Nutrition Reviews 37: 142-144, 1979.

Von Lossonczy, T.O.. et.al., "The effect of a fish diet on lipids in healthy human subjects." American Journal of clinical Nutrition 31: 11340-1346, 1978.

Weisburger, John H., "Dietary fat and risk of chronic disease." Journal of the American Dietetic Association 97, no. 7: S16-S23, 1997.

White, P.L., and Selvy, N. "Let's talk about food." Acton, Mass.: Publishing Sciences, 1974.

Williams, R.J., "Nutritional individually." Readings in Health 80/81. Guilford, Conn.: Dushkin Publishing Group, 1980.

Wood, P. California diet and exercise program. Mountain View, Calif.: Anderson World Books, 1983.

Wood, P.D, et. al., "The distribution of plasma lipoproteins in middle-aged male runners," Metabolism 25: 1249-1257, 1976.

Wood, P.D., et al, "Plasma lipoprotein distribution in male and female runners." Annals of the New York Academy of Sciences 301: 748-763, 1977.

Woods, M.N, "Hormonal levels during dietary changes in premenopausal African American women." Journal of the National Cancer Institute 88, no.19: 1369-1374, 1996.

Zelinski, M.R., Muenchow, M., Wallig, M.A., Horn, P.L., and Woods, J.a. "Exercise delays allogeneic tumor growth and reduces intratumoral inflammation and vascularization." Journal of Applied Physiology 96 (6): 2249-2256. Epub March 12, 2004.

Zuti, W.B., and Golding, L.A. Comparing diet and exercise as weight reduction tools. The physician and Sportsmedicine 4 (1): 49-53, 1973.

978-0-595-47811-8
0-595-47811-5

www.ingramcontent.com/pod-product-compliance
Lightning Source LLC
Chambersburg PA
CBHW030256290526
45785CB00001B/110